To my husband, Greg.

C'est le ton qui fait la chanson.

It's the melody that makes the song.

FUNDAMENTALS

OF

SPORT AND EXERCISE NUTRITION

 Human Kinetics' Fundamentals of Sport and Exercise Science Series

Marie Dunford, PhD, RD

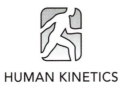

HUMAN KINETICS

Library of Congress Cataloging-in-Publication Data

Dunford, Marie.
  Fundamentals of sport and exercise nutrition / Marie Dunford.
    p. ; cm. -- (Human Kinetics' fundamentals of sport and exercise science series)
  Includes bibliographical references and index.
  ISBN-13: 978-0-7360-7631-9 (soft cover)
  ISBN-10: 0-7360-7631-X (soft cover)
  1. Athletes--Nutrition. 2. Physical fitness--Nutritional aspects . I. Title. II. Series: Fundamentals of sport and exercise science series.
  [DNLM: 1. Nutritional Physiological Phenomena. 2. Exercise--physiology. 3. Sports--physiology. QT 260 D915f 2010]
  TX361.A8D857 2010
  613.2'024796--dc22

2009025712

ISBN-10: 0-7360-7631-X
ISBN-13: 978-0-7360-7631-9

QT 260 D915f 2010
Dunford, Marie.
Fundamentals of sport and exercise
nutrition /....
10030355

Copyright © 2010 by Marie Dunford

The Web addresses cited in this text were current as of July 2009, unless otherwise noted.

Acquisitions Editor: Michael S. Bahrke, PhD; **Developmental Editor:** Maggie Schwarzentraub; **Managing Editor:** Katherine Maurer; **Assistant Editors:** Nicole Gleeson and Scott Hawkins; **Copyeditor:** Patsy Fortney; **Proofreader:** Jim Burns; **Indexer:** Betty Frizzell; **Permission Manager:** Dalene Reeder; **Graphic Designer:** Bob Reuther; **Graphic Artist:** Denise Lowry; **Cover Designer:** Bob Reuther; **Photographer (interior):** © Human Kinetics unless otherwise noted.; **Photo Asset Manager:** Laura Fitch; **Visual Production Assistant:** Joyce Brumfield; **Photo Production Manager:** Jason Allen; **Art Manager:** Kelly Hendren; **Associate Art Manager:** Alan L. Wilborn; **Illustrator:** Tammy Page; **Printer:** McNaughton & Gunn

Printed in the United States of America   10 9 8 7 6 5 4 3 2 1

The paper in this book is certified under a sustainable forestry program.

Human Kinetics
Web site: www.HumanKinetics.com

United States: Human Kinetics, P.O. Box 5076, Champaign, IL 61825-5076
800-747-4457
e-mail: humank@hkusa.com

Canada: Human Kinetics, 475 Devonshire Road Unit 100, Windsor, ON N8Y 2L5
800-465-7301 (in Canada only)
e-mail: info@hkcanada.com

Europe: Human Kinetics, 107 Bradford Road, Stanningley, Leeds LS28 6AT, United Kingdom
+44 (0) 113 255 5665
e-mail: hk@hkeurope.com

Australia: Human Kinetics, 57A Price Avenue, Lower Mitcham, South Australia 5062
08 8372 0999
e-mail: info@hkaustralia.com

New Zealand: Human Kinetics, P.O. Box 80, Torrens Park, South Australia 5062
0800 222 062
e-mail: info@hknewzealand.com

E4629

Contents

Series Preface

The sport sciences have matured impressively over the past 40 years. Subdisciplines in kinesiology have established their own rigorous paths of research, and physical education in its many forms is now an accepted discipline in higher education. Our need now is not only for comprehensive resources that contain all the knowledge that the field has acquired, but also for resources that summarize the foundations of each of the sport sciences for the variety of people who make use of that information today. Understanding the basic topics, goals, and applications of the subdisciplines in kinesiology is critical for students and professionals in many walks of life. Human Kinetics has developed the Fundamentals of Sport and Exercise Science series with these needs in mind.

This and the other books in the series will not provide you with all the in-depth knowledge required for earning an advanced degree or for opening a practice in this subject area. This book will not make you an expert on the subject. What this book will do is give you an excellent grounding in the key themes, terms, history, and status of the subject in both the academic and professional worlds. You can use this grounding as a jumping-off point for studying more in-depth resources and for generating questions for more experienced people in the field. We've even included an annotated list of additional resources for you to consult as you continue your journey.

You might be using this book to help you improve your professional skills or to assess the potential job market. You might want to learn about a new subject, supplement a textbook, or introduce a colleague or client to this exciting subject area. In any of these cases, this book will be your guide to the basics of this subject. It is succinct, informative, and entertaining. You will begin the book with many questions, and you will surely finish it with many more questions. But they will be more thoughtful, complex, substantive questions. We hope that you will use this book to help the sport sciences, and this subject in particular, continue to prosper for another generation.

Key to Icons

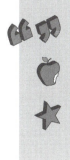

Look for the giant quotation marks, which set off noteworthy quotes from researchers and professionals in the field.

Nutrition Bites include quirky or surprising "Did you know?" types of information.

Success Stories highlight influential individuals in the field. Through these sidebars, you will learn how researchers and professionals apply their knowledge of the subject to their work, and you'll be able to explore possible career paths in the field.

Preface

Fundamentals of Sport and Exercise Nutrition is an introduction to the exciting world of nutrition as a way to enhance training, speed recovery, and reach peak performance. Nutrition is a relatively new field, just over a hundred years old, and sport and exercise nutrition is very new, coming into its own in the 1980s. More research is being conducted and many new products are being created to help athletes improve training and reach peak performance. Athletes are bombarded with information about performance-enhancing supplements. A few of these supplements, such as creatine, may be helpful to some athletes, but many are unproven or not effective. Some supplements are even contaminated with banned substances.

Sport and exercise nutrition is on the cutting edge, a very exciting place to be. But sometimes it can be a confusing place. Because nutrition is a young scientific field, information can be contradictory, incomplete, or nonexistent. For example, what is the best weight loss diet? Some say it should be low in fat, whereas others say it should be low in carbohydrate. How does this debate apply to athletes who need sufficient carbohydrate daily to be able to train and don't want to lose muscle mass in the process of dieting? These questions cannot be answered definitively, but there is sufficient information to make sound recommendations while more research is completed.

Additionally, the application of the information is not always easy. Should an athlete drink water or a sport beverage? Which is a better snack—a high-protein bar or a high-carbohydrate bar? Will supplement X enhance performance? The answers to these questions depend on the situation. For example, if the athlete needs only fluid, then water is an appropriate beverage. However, if both fluid and carbohydrate are needed, then a sport beverage is the better choice.

If you need more information about sport and exercise nutrition, then *Fundamentals of Sport and Exercise Nutrition* will be an invaluable resource. It is an overview of the subject matter and provides a mix of current evidence and the application of that information to athletes in various sports. It is written to inform, enlighten, and inspire further investigation. Each chapter summarizes the current body of knowledge and practice and can be used as a reference by athletes, those who work with athletes, students, and instructors who touch on sport and exercise nutrition in their courses.

The primary purpose of the book is to present introductory information about the field of sport and exercise nutrition. Part I is an introduction to and history of the field. It clarifies some of the terminology used such as exercise nutrition, sport nutrition, and sport dietitian. The first chapter answers a very basic question: What is sport and exercise nutrition? Chapter 2 discusses sport nutrition on a more personal level by exploring what you can do in this exciting field. It talks about the kinds of jobs available in sport nutrition and the education necessary for

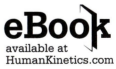

available at
HumanKinetics.com

ix

those jobs. You may want to become a board-certified sport dietitian and counsel competitive athletes.

Part II of the book summarizes current sport nutrition knowledge. It begins with an explanation of energy balance and imbalance in chapter 3. A very simple but important concept is "energy in" (food) and "energy out" (metabolism and exercise). The six chapters that follow are devoted to each of the six essential nutrients—carbohydrate, protein, fat, vitamins, minerals, and water. These nutrients are the heart of sport nutrition.

The nutrients themselves are important, but any book about sport nutrition would fall short without extensive coverage of body weight, body composition, and performance. These are addressed in chapter 10. Body weight is particularly important for athletes whose weight needs to be certified, such as wrestlers and boxers. However, for most athletes weight is a reflection of something much more important to performance—body composition. In many sports, athletes try to attain a relatively high percentage of muscle and a relatively low percentage of body fat. The most appropriate competitive weight and body composition is influenced by the sport or the position played and the athlete's genetic predisposition to leanness.

Unfortunately, in the quest to reach a certain weight or body composition, an athlete may become overly restrictive and obsessed with food intake. Normal eating can become disordered and, eventually, can result in an eating disorder such as anorexia or bulimia. Anyone who works with athletes must be aware of the warning signs and intervene as soon as possible. The final chapter addresses these issues and also explains the female athlete triad. The female athlete triad involves three interrelated factors unique to female athletes: energy availability, menstrual function, and bone mineral density.

Information about dietary supplements is integrated throughout the chapters. This organization is intentional because questions about supplements naturally flow from discussions of essential nutrients and energy balance. Supplementation is complementary to, not exclusive of, dietary intake, so it makes sense to address food and supplements at the same time. For example, a discussion of the nutrient protein would be incomplete without addressing protein supplements. Many supplements are marketed to athletes to help them enhance their energy levels, lose weight, and increase muscle mass quickly, and all of these issues are addressed.

This book includes user-friendly features. Each chapter begins with a list of objectives and ends with a list of summary points. Numerous boxes highlight interesting topics, myths, and popular beliefs. Each chapter features a person who has been successful in the field of sport and exercise nutrition.

Fundamentals of Sport and Exercise Nutrition is a summary of the essential issues related to sport and exercise nutrition. The scientific information has been distilled, not diluted, and the application of this information naturally follows. The book is written for those who want to improve their knowledge and understanding of an important aspect of sport performance and exercise training. You can feel confident about your understanding of the field of sport and exercise nutrition with this one-stop, go-to resource!

Acknowledgments

I would like to thank Mike Bahrke, acquisitions editor, not only for contacting me about writing this book, but also for providing a steady hand during its development. Maggie Schwarzentraub is a skilled and understanding developmental editor. Thanks for giving me enough rope to do my job but not enough to hang myself. Special thanks to my colleagues who agreed to be featured in the success stories in each chapter. Sport and exercise nutrition has come into its own because of such dedicated people, and each of you is an inspiration. To all those named and unnamed, thank you for your contributions to this book.

I
PART

Welcome to Sport and Exercise Nutrition

Part I consists of two chapters that introduce the field of sport and exercise nutrition. Chapter 1 begins with a history and includes a time line. Sport nutrition emerged from the fields of nutrition and exercise physiology and maintains a close relationship with these fields today. However, sport nutrition and exercise physiology have developed into separate disciplines.

Each field related to athletics, whether it is nutrition, exercise physiology, or training, has developed to the point at which there are recognized credentials for those who work in that field. Chapter 2 explains the kinds of jobs available in the growing field of sport nutrition and the credential needed to be a sport dietitian. The chapter also explains about scope of practice and how to know the limits of professional training. In many cases, if you work with athletes, you need to know about sport nutrition because you are involved with coaching or training. However, if sport nutrition is not your primary area of expertise, you must also know when to refer an athlete to someone with more specific training.

CHAPTER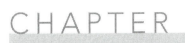

What Is Sport and Exercise Nutrition?

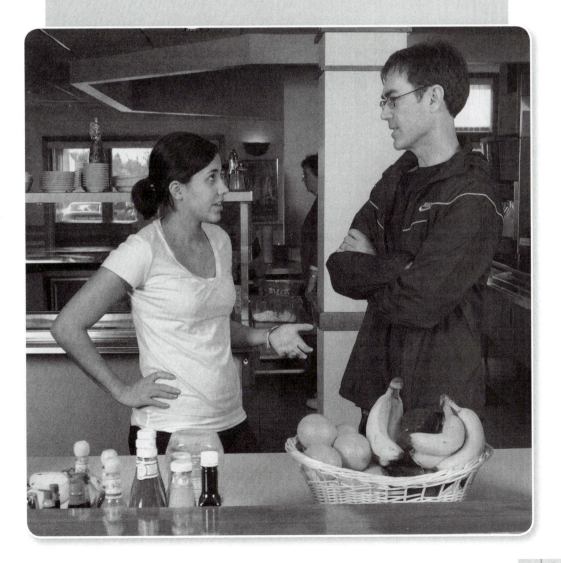

"To eat is a necessity, but to eat intelligently is an art."

Francois de la Rochefoucauld,
French author (1613-1680)

At the 1904 Olympics held in St. Louis, Thomas Hicks won the gold medal in the marathon. The race was run in temperatures near 32 °C (89.6 °F), and there were only two places along the route for water. At the 30-kilometer mark (18.6 miles), he asked for water but received a wet sponge to suck on and the white of an egg. A few kilometers later, nearing collapse, he received two eggs, a sip of brandy, and a small dose of strychnine (erroneously thought to be a stimulant and later used as a rat poison). Over the final 2 kilometers that included two hills, he was given two more eggs and two more shots of brandy, purportedly one for each hill. He finished the race but was unable to receive his trophy because he was in medical distress. So much for the prevailing advice on sport nutrition at the time!

Sport nutrition, which can also be called exercise nutrition, is the application of nutrition principles for the purpose of improving training, recovery, and performance. Exercise nutrition is a logical name for this discipline because it also reflects the close relationship between the academic fields of **exercise physiology** and nutrition. However, the field is much more commonly called sport nutrition. Sports are competitive physical activities, although the term is being expanded to include other competitions (interestingly, poker tournaments are now being covered in the sports section of some newspapers). Although *exercise nutrition* is perhaps a better term, *sport nutrition* is likely to remain the most widely used term and is used throughout this book.

sport nutrition—The study of nutrition for the purpose of improving training, recovery, and performance.

exercise physiology—The study of how the body adapts to exercise.

Origins and History of Sport Nutrition

Athletes have always been advised about what to eat, but the academic field now known as sport nutrition began in the exercise physiology laboratories. Historians consider the first studies of sport nutrition to be those of carbohydrate and fat metabolism conducted in Sweden in the late 1930s. In the late 1960s Scandinavian scientists began to study muscle glycogen storage, use, and resynthesis associated with prolonged exercise. Technology was also developed to help those scientists measure human tissue responses to exercise. In 1965 something else was born in the laboratory. At the University of Florida a team of researchers led by Dr. Robert Cade developed a scientifically formulated beverage for the school's football team. It bears his name and that of the school's mascot—Gatorade.

In the 1970s exercise physiologists worldwide, but particularly in the United States, began to develop exercise physiology laboratories at universities and to study trained athletes. Distance runners and cyclists were most frequently studied because these athletes were in danger of depleting their glycogen stores and these sports could be simulated easily in the laboratory with the use of treadmills and stationary bikes. Research facilities at military and astronaut training centers also were developed because these individuals need to be in top physical condition. Much of the initial published research focused on the use of carbohydrate.

Some research on protein was conducted, but studying protein was much more difficult than studying carbohydrate because protein is found in so many different places in the body. Body-builders were particularly interested in knowing more about how to obtain the maximum amount of protein and the highest rate of protein synthesis in skeletal muscles, but there was little research to answer their questions. Some scientists questioned whether

Nutrition Bite

Athletes have always been given advice about what to eat, some of which seems rather odd today. Here is a sample:

- In the ancient Olympics, eating goat meat was advised because it was thought to confer strength.
- Athletes in ancient Greece were advised to eat dried figs as part of their training diet.
- Milo of Croton, a five-time ancient Olympic wrestling champion, reportedly ate 20 pounds (9 kg) of meat, 20 pounds (9 kg) of bread, and 18 pints (8.5 l) of wine a day, although such an intake would be impossible.
- Brandy drinking was a marathon race strategy at the 1904 and 1908 Olympics.
- When Mary Decker (Slaney) was smashing track records as a teenager in the 1970s, her admission that she ate a plate of spaghetti the night before a race brought surprise and laughter from the press.

1910-1929

1913
First vitamin (vitamin A) is discovered in the laboratory.

1917
The American Dietetic Association is established to improve public health.

1919
Harris and Benedict publish a study about basal metabolism in man.

1927
The Harvard Fatigue Lab is established. The lab's work is at the forefront of the field of exercise physiology.

1929
Nobel Prize is awarded to Frederick Hopkins and Christiaan Eijkman for the discovery of vitamins.

1930-1949

1937
Hans Krebs discovers the citric acid cycle, eventually known as the Krebs cycle. In the 1950s he receives a Nobel Prize and is knighted for his work.

1938-1939
Carbohydrate and fat metabolism studies are conducted in Stockholm. These are considered the first studies in sport nutrition.

1941
Establishment of nutrient intake standards in the United States, known as the Recommended Dietary Allowances (RDAs)

1945
Albert Behnke and colleagues devise an underwater weighing system for measuring body composition. It is the standard for almost 40 years.

1950-1969

1950
Keys and colleagues publish groundbreaking work on human starvation.

1954
American College of Sports Medicine is founded.

1956
Siri equation for determining body composition is published.

1965
Gatorade is created at the University of Florida.

1966-1967
Bergstrom and colleagues publish groundbreaking studies linking diet, muscle glycogen, and physical performance.

(continued)

bodybuilding was a sport; many considered it more of a sideshow compared to other athletic competitions. For these and other reasons, bodybuilders began to learn about nutrition via personal experimentation and trial and error. Although there is more research on protein today, many of the fundamental questions about the amount and timing of protein intake remain because of the difficulty of studying these subjects. The optimal amount of protein intake for athletes continues to be a controversial subject.

As is the case with much laboratory research, knowledge leads to application. This resulted in more collaboration between exercise physiologists and nutritionists, particularly beginning in the 1980s. For example, exercise physiologists were discovering that endurance athletes, such as marathon runners and long-distance cyclists, benefited from consuming approximately 8 grams of carbohydrate per kilogram of body weight daily. But what food and beverages did athletes need to eat to obtain this much carbohydrate? Would such a high-carbohydrate diet meet the body's other nutritional needs to maintain good health? The expertise of nutritionists was needed for translating scientific information into practical applications.

The 1980s marked the emergence of the field known as sport nutrition. Considering its importance in supporting excellent athletic performance, sport nutrition as a specialized discipline developed relatively late. Initially, much of the focus was on endurance athletes, which paralleled the exercise physiology research that was being conducted. In fact, athletes were typically characterized as either endurance or strength athletes. Endurance athletes often focused primarily on carbohydrate intake; strength athletes focused primarily on protein intake.

> *Sports nutrition didn't exist when I began college. My great fortune was to find a wonderful lecturer, passionate scientist, and keen runner—Professor Richard Read. At dinner I noticed he was only eating lettuce and cheese in preparation for a marathon. He had read some recently published papers about a diet that could help store more muscle glycogen. I was hooked. Sports nutrition was just evolving and I could see it happen before my eyes.*
>
> **Louise Burke**, PhD, APD, sport nutrition pioneer based in Australia

During this time tremendous advances were being made in the training of athletes. By the 1990s resistance training was becoming a part of nearly all training and conditioning programs, including those for endurance athletes. Many predominantly strength athletes were beginning to incorporate more aerobic activities into their training. Strength athletes more carefully considered their carbohydrate intake, and endurance athletes were more thoughtful about their protein intake. Athletes also began to train harder and for longer periods than in the past. Nutrition was widely recognized as a way to support training and speed recovery. It became clear that the intensity and duration of training were major influences on athletes' nutritional needs.

But training is not the end point for athletes—performance is. Thus, athletes also needed to know what to eat before, during, and immediately after performance. Choosing the wrong foods or beverages before or during competition can be disastrous. Some sports, such as wrestling and boxing, require weight to be certified. If the time of the scheduled weigh-in is rapidly approaching, these athletes may try to alter their weight by inducing fluid loss or excessive sweating, strategies that can endanger both performance and health. Poor nutritional planning can result in the inability to compete or perform well.

The mid-1990s added another dimension to the field of sport nutrition—dietary supplements. In 1994 the Dietary Supplement Health and Education Act deregulated dietary supplements in the United States. The act also classified herbs and botanicals as dietary supplements and included them in the same category as vitamin, mineral, and amino acid (protein) supplements. However, because some of these herbs are stimulants, classifying them as dietary supplements has caused problems. For example, the herb

Nutrition Bite

Here are some nutrition facts that will give you food for thought:

- **Protein supplements typically contain the same kinds of protein found in milk, meat, fish, poultry, eggs, and soy.** Food and supplements are not mutually exclusive; rather, they are complementary. Thus, dietary supplements should be considered in the context of the athlete's overall nutrition plan.

- **Energy beverages typically are high in sugar and caffeine.** A highly sugared drink raises blood sugar quickly, and caffeine is a stimulant, which is why these drinks help athletes feel energetic. But the effects of both subside rather quickly, leaving the athlete in need of another energy fix.

- **Some granola bars are high in fat and low in fiber but can be advertised as "healthy."** Do some detective work by reading the ingredient label to get some idea of how granola bars differ. Any company can use the word *healthy* to describe its product.

- **A sweet potato has more carbohydrate and fiber than a white potato.** Variety is the spice of life. Why not include both in your diet?

1970-1989

1971
David Costill's lab studies the usage and synthesis of muscle glycogen during prolonged exercise on successive days. Such studies help establish how much carbohydrate endurance athletes need daily.

1972
Low-carbohydrate diets become popular with the publication of the book *Dr. Atkins' Diet Revolution*.

1978
Caffeine is suggested to improve endurance performance both in the scientific literature and the popular magazine *Runner's World*. Athletes are beginning to look to scientists for ways to improve performance.

1981
David Jenkins, a Canadian physician and nutrition professor at the University of Toronto, Canada, publishes an article on the effect of dietary carbohydrate on blood glucose. Known as the glycemic index, it becomes an important tool for diabetics and athletes.

Sports, Cardiovascular, and Wellness Nutritionists (SCAN), a subgroup of the American Dietetic Association, is established.

1983
Jack Wilmore publishes information about the body composition of athletes in various sports.

Phinney and colleagues publish a study suggesting that a high-fat, extremely low-carbohydrate diet could improve the performance of endurance athletes such as distance cyclists. Subsequent studies show that such diets are not beneficial to performance.

1985
Timothy Noakes, a South African professor of exercise and sport science, first reports a case of hyponatremia (low blood sodium) in a female distance runner. Overconsumption of water, known as water intoxication, is a likely cause.

Barbara Drinkwater's lab reports differences in bone mineral content between menstruating and nonmenstruating female athletes.

1987
Brown, Steen, and Wilmore analyze weight regulation practices in wrestlers and the effects they have on metabolism.

(continued)

ephedra has a much narrower safe dose range than other dietary supplements and has been implicated in some athletes' deaths. The law does not require dietary supplement manufacturers to prove safety and effectiveness before their supplements are marketed (as is the case with over-the-counter and prescription medications). The 1994 act led to the direct marketing of dietary supplements to consumers with little government oversight, and athletes became a prime target.

★ SUCCESS STORY

Bob Seebohar, Fuel4mance and Elite Triathlon Coach

Bob Seebohar, MS, RD, CSSD, CSCS, lives and breathes sport nutrition. He is a sport dietitian, professional endurance coach, author, and ultraendurance athlete. Bob turned a personal passion into a professional passion! He studied exercise physiology as an undergraduate, spent three years working as a wellness specialist and fitness professional, and then pursued two graduate degrees studying exercise physiology and metabolism and nutrition. When asked if you need that much education, he replied, "You can learn how to work with an athlete in a field setting, but you cannot learn the foundation knowledge without formal education. This knowledge provides you the confidence to work with athletes of all ages, types, and abilities and should not be overlooked. Formal education teaches you the background information required to successfully plan, develop, and implement athletes' performance nutrition plans while in the field."

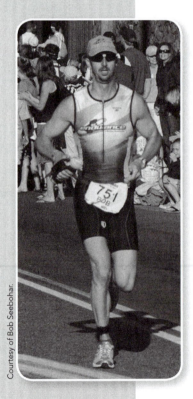

Courtesy of Bob Seebohar.

Bob formed a path that allowed him to work with the best of the best from endurance to collegiate and Olympic-caliber athletes. He believes that personal participation in athletics is crucial for being successful in the sport nutrition field. Many thought that he would not be able to relate well with college football players because he is an endurance athlete. However, his athletic accomplishments helped the players feel confident that he knew what he was talking about and that he indeed practiced what he preached. He gained their respect first through his athleticism, which allowed him to then show his sport nutrition expertise as it related to improving their performance. You don't need to be an elite athlete to be a sport dietitian, but you must understand the principles of sport.

Bob has advice for those who want a career in sport nutrition: "Engage and surround yourself with the best. Be well read and ask questions. Choose a couple of mentors whom you can learn from and who will help to guide your journey. Be willing to think and operate outside the box. Hold to your values and do not compromise your integrity but be willing to explore the vast opportunities that are present in this field. Keep up with the research and the in-field practices that athletes do or you will get left behind and your credibility will diminish."

The use of dietary supplements is an integral part of sport nutrition. It is estimated that 75 to 90 percent of college and professional athletes use dietary supplements, usually vitamins, minerals, and creatine (McDowall, 2007). Such high use may influence younger aspiring athletes to take dietary supplements. These are the fundamental questions that any athlete should ask about a dietary supplement: Is it legal? Is it ethical? Is it safe? Is it effective? Overall, only a handful of dietary supplements have been proven to be effective.

In the fields of medicine, exercise physiology, and nutrition, the 2000s have been marked by the emergence of **evidence-based recommendations**. *Evidence-based* refers to the use of scientific research to determine effectiveness. In the past, recommendations have been based not only on scientific evidence but also on consensus of opinion and historical practice. Evidence-based recommendations require that sufficient high-quality research be conducted so that unbiased conclusions about effectiveness can be drawn. The time line summarizes the development of the field of sport nutrition.

> **evidence-based recommendations**—Recommendations based on scientific studies of effectiveness.

Sport Nutrition as a Subspecialty of Nutrition

Sport nutrition is a specialized field of nutrition that takes into account the demands of training and performance, but it always builds on sound principles of nutrition. Like all humans, athletes must meet basic nutritional needs to remain in good health and recover from injury and illness. Nutrition and exercise are two major factors in good health, so athletes are wise to routinely eat a healthful diet even when they are not training.

General nutrition guidelines need to be modified to support training, recovery, and performance. In the long term, those goals are met by adequate energy, nutrient, and fluid intake. Short-term goals typically involve specific changes to the diet such as the amount and timing of food and fluid intake. Nutrition standards and guidelines developed for the general population are useful tools, especially for recreational and novice athletes, but the demands of rigorous exercise training and competition require specific dietary modifications.

Athletes have widely accepted the need for well-designed training and conditioning programs but have been slower to adopt the dietary strategies that support training. Athletes are recognizing

1970-1989
(continued)

1988
Ivy and colleagues report the effect of various amounts of dietary carbohydrate on muscle glycogen synthesis. Such studies result in specific guidelines for carbohydrate intake for endurance athletes.

1990 TO PRESENT

1992
An association between disordered eating, amenorrhea, and osteoporosis in female athletes in sports that emphasize a lean physique is reported. This condition is called the female athlete triad.

1993
Texas Woman's University begins offering a master's degree in exercise and sport nutrition.

1994
The U.S. Congress passes the Dietary Supplement Health and Education Act, which deregulates dietary supplements. Athletes become a target for supplement advertising.

1997
The Dietary Reference Intakes (DRI) incorporate the Recommended Dietary Allowances (RDA) and become the new system for nutrient guidelines for the United States and Canada.

Three collegiate wrestlers die as a result of intentional rapid weight loss, prompting a reexamination of practices used in cutting weight.

1999
Low-carbohydrate diets again become popular with the publication of the book *Dr. Atkins' New Diet Revolution*.

2004
The American College of Sports Medicine publishes position stands on exercise and fluid replacement and exertional heat illness during training and competition.

2007
The American College of Sports Medicine updates its position paper on the female athlete triad.

2009
Nutrition and Athletic Performance Position Paper is published by the American Dietetic Association, Dietitians of Canada, and the American College of Sports Medicine. It provides comprehensive information about sport nutrition.

the advantages associated with following sport nutrition recommendations and not leaving their dietary intake to chance. Those who aspire to be professionals cannot afford to overlook any aspect that may result in top performance. Professional and college athletes today face longer seasons than in the past and nearly year-round training. Many professional athletes wish to continue to compete into their 30s and 40s. Proper nutrition is crucial and may make the difference between winning and losing or playing and retirement.

> *Bodybuilding is much like any other sport. To be successful you must dedicate yourself 100% to your training, diet, and mental approach.*
>
> **Arnold Schwarzenegger**, former Mr. Olympia (1970-1975), elected governor of California in 2003

Is Sport Nutrition an Art or a Science?

Sport nutrition is both an art and a science. At the core, exercise physiology and nutrition are scientific fields and both have well-established links to medicine. Sport nutrition recommendations are based on scientific research. But applying the results of research studies to individual athletes is an art that takes skill and judgment.

Eating is not solely physiological, and people are not robots that are fed pre-scribed formulas. Rather, people select food based on their likes and dislikes. Food provides the nutrients that people need, but obtaining nutrients is not the only reason people eat. Likewise, food consumption is influenced not only by hunger, but also by psychological, social, cultural, and religious factors. There is no perfect diet or one dietary pattern that all people should follow.

Even well-tested scientific principles have to be adapted to the individual. Scientific studies have shown that carbohydrate intake during prolonged endurance exercise, such as long-distance running, cycling, and swimming, can improve performance by delaying the onset of fatigue. But the application of this principle varies among athletes in the same sport. For example, one marathon runner may prefer to consume only a carbohydrate-containing sport beverage, whereas another prefers a carbohydrate gel and water. A third marathoner may alternate a carbohydrate food with a sport beverage. The science behind the behavior is the same, but applying that science is an art. Sport nutritionists do not tell athletes what to eat. They assess current food intake, help athletes set goals, and counsel them on how to reach their goals by discussing all the possible options.

The Short of It

- Sport nutrition and exercise physiology are closely tied.
- The goals of sport nutrition are to help athletes improve training, recovery, and performance while maintaining good health.

- Rigorous training taxes the body, and proper foods and fluids are needed for recovery.
- Sport nutrition recommendations are based on science, but putting those recommendations into practice is an art.
- Athletes should not leave their diets to chance.

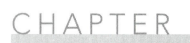

CHAPTER **2**

What Can I Do With Sport Nutrition?

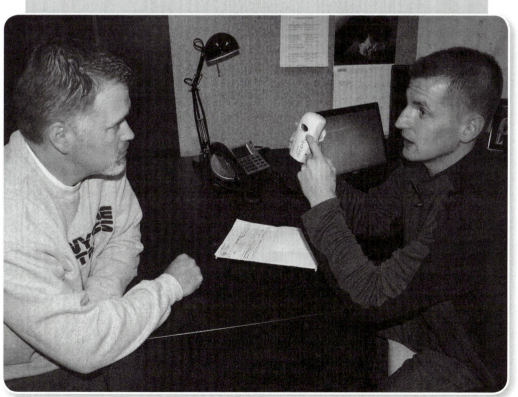

Courtesy of Mark Daly.

In this chapter, you will learn the following:

✓ The kinds of jobs available in sport nutrition
✓ The credentials required for becoming a sport dietitian
✓ How sport nutrition fits into other sport-related professions

"Exercise is king. Nutrition is queen. Put them together and you've got a kingdom!"

Jack LaLanne, fitness legend who celebrated his 70th birthday by swimming 1.5 miles (2.4 km) towing 70 boats with 70 people while handcuffed and shackled

Sport nutritionists are a diverse group working in any number of challenging settings, including sports medicine clinics, universities, conditioning facilities, and fitness clubs. Some are practitioners who own and operate home-based consulting businesses. Despite these career options, many people do not know what sport nutritionists do on a daily basis, especially practitioners who own their own practices. Here is a glance at a day in the life of Brian Zehetner, a registered dietitian (RD), board-certified specialist in sports dietetics (CSSD), and certified strength and conditioning specialist (CSCS). Brian works with golfers, ultimate fighters, boxers, and endurance athletes and currently consults with the Milwaukee Bucks of the NBA. He also works with numerous NHL players and is a nationally known sport nutrition writer.

Brian gets up early and starts his day by checking e-mails and catching up on phone messages. He also schedules appointments and sends out invoices before heading out to meet with clients at their places of work, local coffee shops, or training facilities. The mornings are ideal for resting metabolic rate tests and initial consultations with prospective clients. The late morning to early afternoon is typically reserved for freelance writing, which involves completing articles for national magazines and moderating nutrition and fitness–related Web sites. By late afternoon, Brian heads back out to meet with individual athletes and clients referred from one of the well-established sports medicine clinics in the area. These appointments finish around 6 p.m., but the workday is not necessarily done. Some of the evening hours may be dedicated to completing assessments and evaluations, finishing any number of nutrition- or fitness-related consulting projects, or managing the business side of the company. Though Brian's workdays often follow the same pattern, the projects, writing assignments, and clients are different almost every day. This varied and flexible schedule is a perfect fit for Brian and his family.

What Jobs Are Associated With Sport Nutrition?

Because sport nutrition is an emerging field, the jobs associated with it are also emerging. Opportunities for full-time positions in sport nutrition are increasing but are still few. Opportunities, in part, depend on the credentials the practitioner holds, which are discussed in more detail in the next section.

Perhaps the most coveted jobs are those involving elite athletes, such as at Olympic training centers, with professional teams, or at universities or training facilities for athletes who hope to become professionals or highly competitive amateurs. For example, the Australian Institute of Sport employs eight **sport dietitians**. The U.S. Olympic Committee also employs full-time sport dietitians, but the number varies between one and four.

> **sport dietitian**—A registered dietitian who is also board certified in sport dietetics.

Professional teams in the United States, Australia, and Western Europe hire sport dietitians, but usually not as full-time employees. In the United States, nearly all of the 32 teams in the National Football League (NFL) hire sport nutrition consultants, but just a few currently have a full-time position. Only a handful of professional basketball, baseball, and hockey teams hire a **sport nutritionist**, and those that do typically hire on a part-time basis. These are exciting jobs, but because consulting jobs are not usually full-time, these sport dietitians are also typically in private practice or hold university or other positions.

> **sport nutritionist**—A general term for someone who applies nutrition information to athletes.

Training centers for elite athletes hoping to become professionals represent another opportunity for sport dietitians. One such center currently employs five sport dietitians, and this number is likely to grow slowly. Individual nutrition counseling is an integral and central part of each athlete's training and conditioning program. Such centers are also expanding to include highly ranked amateurs and other recreational athletes who are serious about improving performance and may result in some additional full-time sport nutrition positions.

Currently, about 65 registered dietitians (RD) practice full- or part-time in collegiate settings, and this number is expected to increase (Ingrid Skoog, MS, RD, CSSD, Department of Nutrition and Exercise Sciences, Oregon State University, personal communication, 2009). In 1996 there were only three full-time collegiate sport nutrition positions. Today there are 15 full-time positions, and most of these people hold the CSSD credential. At least 50 universities hire sport nutritionists on a part-time basis. Although not exclusive to athletes, nutrition counseling by RDs is usually available through student health centers.

Some sport nutritionists are self-employed and have full- or part-time private practices in which they counsel a range of clients from professionals to those aspiring to be collegiate or professional athletes to recreational athletes trying to improve their personal best performances. Many private practices are located in metropolitan areas to maintain a large enough client base. Because nutrition is an integral part of athletic training, some sport nutritionists also seek expertise in the area of training, such as becoming a certified strength and conditioning specialist, so they can offer more comprehensive services. For example, a small number of people certified in both disciplines offer private nutrition, training, and conditioning services to dedicated athletes.

Many health and fitness clubs have nutrition services available for their members. These positions are often part-time, and the person is typically an independent contractor, not an employee of the club. Consultation usually takes place at the fitness center. In many cases, the clients are recreational athletes who are more focused on weight loss than on improving performance. Similarly, personal trainers often find themselves training clients who want to increase their fitness and conditioning as well as alter their body composition. Although sport nutrition is not their primary job, it becomes a component of the job because successful weight loss involves both diet and exercise.

What Degrees and Credentials Are Needed?

Recall from chapter 1 that exercise physiology and nutrition began as separate disciplines but became integrated when the focus became athletic training and performance. Therefore, early in the history of the field of sport nutrition, experts had their academic training in either exercise physiology or nutrition. Many of today's leading sport nutritionists have at least a bachelor's degree in exercise physiology, nutrition, or dietetics. However, an undergraduate degree in any one of these fields does not include much cross-disciplinary course work. For example, most exercise physiology programs include one general nutrition class, and dietetics programs require the study of physiology but not exercise physiology.

> *No man ever reached to excellence in any one art or profession without having passed through the slow and painful process of study and preparation.*
>
> **Horace,** Roman poet (65-8 BC)

In the United States approximately 43 colleges and universities offer undergraduate or graduate degrees associated with sport nutrition. At the bachelor's degree level some programs have a sport nutrition track, concentration, or minor associated with an undergraduate degree in nutrition. Most of the 43 offer a master's degree specializing in sport nutrition that includes course work in both exercise science and nutrition. A handful of programs offer a PhD integrating the fields of nutrition and exercise physiology. For a partial listing of sport nutrition education programs, go to www.scandpg.org/sport_nutrition_education_program.php, or check the Web sites of area colleges.

There is no national sport nutrition organization that accredits sport nutrition programs. In contrast, a master's or doctoral degree in physical therapy (there is no BS degree) is offered at almost 200 U.S. universities, all of which are accredited by the American Physical Therapy Association. For those who are beginning their college education, it would be wise to choose a degree program with the greatest opportunity to take sport nutrition course work. For those pursuing an advanced degree, earning one in the area of sport nutrition would be highly recommended. However, the number of programs is limited.

The number of people with a master's or doctoral degree in sport nutrition will increase in the coming decades, and one day those degrees may be preferred or required for jobs in sport nutrition. At the present time there is an effort to certify sport nutritionists. In the health professions, certification is considered the gold standard for quality care. Certification typically requires academic course work, professional experience, mastery of standards of practice, passage of an exam, and ongoing continuing education. Once certification requirements have been met, people can use the official certification designation after their names. The certification requirements can vary depending on the standards set by the organization responsible for the certification.

At the present time the term *sport nutritionist* can be used by anyone regardless of academic training or experience. Thus, when someone claims to be a sport nutritionist, consumers should find out the nature and extent of the training this person has received. A variety of sport nutrition credentials and certificates are described here, but they are not equivalent, and consumers are cautioned to ask more about the training of anyone practicing in the area of sport nutrition.

The American Dietetic Association began offering its Board Certified Specialist in Sports Dietetics (CSSD) in 2006 and more than 300 have earned the CSSD. Sport dietitians are credentialed health professionals, having already obtained their registered dietitian (RD) credential. To be eligible to take the CSSD exam, a person must be a registered dietitian for at least two years and have at least 1,500 hours of experience working with athletes and active individuals. The requirements for becoming an RD include a bachelor's degree, course work in dietetics, completion of a postbaccalaureate internship, and passage of a national exam. In addition to counseling healthy athletes, CSSDs can legally provide medical nutrition therapy because they are registered dietitians. For example, they can counsel athletes with diabetes, high blood pressure, and high blood cholesterol.

Another recent certification is the Certified Sports Nutritionist from the International Society of Sports Nutrition (CISSN). On its Web site, the ISSN suggests that the exam would be difficult to pass without a four-year degree in exercise science, kinesiology, physical education, nutrition, biology, or a related biological science. Those with a four-year degree in a field outside of the biological sciences should complete a one-semester sport nutrition course. However, a person without a four-year degree may take the exam if he or she has been practicing in the field of sport nutrition for at least five years, is a paid member of the ISSN, has attended at least three ISSN meetings in the past four years, is certified as a trainer, and has one certification in nutrition (accepted certifications are listed on the Web site).

Various organizations offer sport nutrition certificates. Certificates are different from certifications. In general, certificates are awarded for the successful completion of a course or series of courses in a particular subject. Most require the passage of an exam as a way to demonstrate knowledge of a subject area. Certificates typically are limited to measuring knowledge, not any other skills that a practitioner should possess.

Some sport nutrition certificates are offered through accredited universities that also offer degrees in nutrition. These certificate programs typically require two prerequisite courses, such as introductory nutrition and physiology, followed by four or five 3-unit (semester units) sport nutrition–related courses. Such certificates are

⭐ SUCCESS STORY

Louise Burke, Australian Institute of Sport

Louise Burke, PhD, APD (accredited practising dietitian), heads the department of sports nutrition at the Australian Institute of Sport (AIS). The AIS was set up in 1981 to revitalize Australian success on the world's sporting stage. The first sport science and medicine positions gave the department of physiology the responsibility to look after athlete nutrition. When the AIS expanded in 1990, Louise Burke was hired.

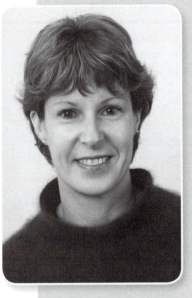

At one level it was a difficult task. However, at another level Louise says it has been easy: "It's always felt like an idea whose time has come! I have been blessed with a dream job, and an incredible team to work with. Of course, along the way I have had to fight for more funding and for support to start new programs or activities. I think that passion and patience are prerequisites for success in equal measure."

Louise Burke competed in Ironman competitions in the mid-1980s; thus, she has personal knowledge of how sport nutrition advice differs today compared to then. "I often tell people that I competed in a previous life. I can't imagine how I had 25 hours a week to ride bikes and run trails, or what I was thinking in choosing to wear leopard-skin trisuits! But the landscape of sport nutrition has also changed so much. When I competed, our bikes had metal toe-clips rather than pedal systems, and the aid stations in Kona served guava jelly sandwiches rather than sport gels. Everything was a challenge requiring a homemade solution and individual trial and error. We learned from top athletes like Dave Scott and Scott Tinley rather than sport scientists. These days, we still recommend that athletes devise an individual nutrition plan, but there are lots of formulas or guidelines to provide a starting point, and lots of tailor-made sport nutrition products to provide the practical help."

In addition to her position at AIS, Louise Burke is a prolific writer, sought-after speaker, editor of the *International Journal of Sport Nutrition and Exercise Metabolism,* and wife and mother.

one way to prepare for certifications that contain a sport nutrition component, such as the American College of Sports Medicine's Health/Fitness Instructor.

Three well-recognized organizations, the American College of Sports Medicine (ACSM), the National Strength and Conditioning Association (NSCA), and the American Council on Exercise (ACE), do not offer certificates or certification in sport nutrition. The majority of sport nutrition certificates appear to be offered by organizations associated with personal trainers. For example, sport nutrition certificates (but not certification) are available through the International Fitness Professionals Association (IFPA), American Fitness Professionals & Associates (AFPA), American Fitness Training of Athletics (AFTA), and the National Federation of Professional Trainers (NFPT). A written manual or workbook is provided as part of the fee to take the exam, and a certificate is earned after passage of the exam. These certificates are often advertised as a way for personal trainers to demonstrate to their clients that they have some formal knowledge of sport nutrition.

Nutrition Bites

The 2009 meeting of the American College of Sports Medicine featured sessions on these hot topics in sport nutrition:

- Sports Nutrition: Lessons from the Beijing Olympic Games
- Vitamin D's Effects on Health and Physical Performance
- Nutraceuticals, Exercise, Health and Performance: Curcumin, Ginger and Quercetin
- Train Low With Carbohydrates—Is There a Case?
- Ramadan: Nutritional Challenges and Solutions for the Muslim Athlete
- Carbohydrate-Protein Supplementation and Endurance Exercise: An Alternative Perspective

How Does Sport Nutrition Interface With Other Professions?

By its nature, sport nutrition is interdisciplinary. As professional sports have grown over the past decades, so too have specialized fields related to sports. In addition to sport nutrition, examples include sports medicine and sport psychology. Practitioners in these fields have their academic training in the primary field, such as medicine, psychology, or nutrition, but have specialized knowledge and experience with sports. They are rightfully seen as experts because of their intimate knowledge of the subject matter. These professionals evaluate and distill the current body of knowledge and make evidence-based recommendations.

Those working directly with athletes must understand the many aspects that can affect athletic performance. For example, a coach must intimately understand the sport as well as the basics of other areas such as training, nutrition, and psychology. Many coaches can help athletes apply the principles of sport nutrition, but most are not experts in the field of sport nutrition. Likewise, many sport-related professionals are asked about nutrition, although this is not their primary area of expertise. For example, certified strength and conditioning specialists (CSCS), certified athletic trainers (ATC), and personal trainers frequently are asked to provide sport nutrition information directly to athletes. How far should a sport-related professional go in providing sport nutrition information?

Everyone wins with good nutrition.

Nancy Clark, MS, RD, CSSD, in her best-selling book *Nancy Clark's Sports Nutrition Guidebook*

Because of sport nutrition's interdisciplinary nature, the boundaries between various disciplines are often not clearly defined. For example, both exercise physiologists and sport nutritionists are concerned about carbohydrate but their expertise and focus are different. Athletes can be harmed by misinformation, so professional limits are important for both the athlete and the practitioner (who could be subject to a malpractice lawsuit).

The delineation of professional boundaries is referred to as **scope of practice.**

scope of practice—The legal and ethical scope of work based on academic training, knowledge, and experience.

Scope of practice refers to the accepted activities, skills, and responsibilities of a practitioner and is based on academic training and experience. Scope of practice protects consumers from practitioners with inadequate training. But it also protects professionals by helping them avoid areas where they are inadequately trained and keeping them from getting in over their heads. When the athlete's need is beyond the practitioner's scope of practice, then the appropriate course of action is to refer the athlete to a professional with that training.

For example, the National Strength and Conditioning Association (NSCA) defines the scope of practice of a certified strength and conditioning specialist as follows: "[to] conduct sports-specific testing sessions, design and implement safe and effective strength training and conditioning programs and provide guidance regarding nutrition and injury prevention." As part of this statement NSCA affirms, "CSCSs consult with and refer athletes to other professionals when appropriate."

State law may define scope of practice. For example, physicians in all states must have a license, and practicing medicine without a license is a criminal offense. Some (but not all) states require licensure for those who work with athletes, such as certified athletic trainers, but at this time no state defines the scope of practice of a sport nutritionist. Knowing and respecting the scope of practice protects athletes and professionals alike.

The Short of It

Sport nutrition is an up-and-coming field.

- Jobs in sport nutrition are currently few but the number is growing.
- Anyone can call himself a sport nutritionist, so consumers should ask about the person's training.
- A special credential is needed to be a sport dietitian.
- Practitioners whose clients' needs are beyond their scope of practice should refer them to professionals with the proper training.

II
PART

Building Blocks of Sport and Exercise Nutrition

Part II contains nine chapters that cover the fundamental topics related to sport nutrition. As is the case with most books that focus on athletes, the first chapter in this part, chapter 3, is about energy. This sets the stage for a discussion of three energy-containing nutrients—carbohydrate, protein, and fat—in chapters 4, 5, and 6. Many athletes do not consume enough carbohydrate in their diets, and their training, recovery, and performance suffer. Protein is always a hot topic with athletes because of its fundamental role in building and maintaining muscle. Unfortunately, many people, including athletes, perceive fat negatively. Fat is a complicated topic because it affects health, body composition, and performance.

The nutrients that do not contain calories—vitamins, minerals, and water—are just as important to athletes as those that do contain calories. These nutrients are discussed in chapters 7, 8, and 9. Without the proper amount of vitamins and minerals, athletes can undermine their training. They can also develop diseases that hamper performance, such as iron-deficiency anemia. One of the biggest influences on performance, especially in the heat, is taking in the right amount of water. Too great a degree of dehydration negatively affects performance and health, but too much water intake can also be dangerous. Water balance depends on sodium and potassium, too, so there is much to be covered in the chapter on water and electrolytes.

Chapter 10 addresses weight, body composition, and performance. Under normal circumstances, athletes are concerned with their scale weight as well as their body composition—that is, the amount and ratio of fat and lean tissues. Chapter 10 summarizes the various methods used to determine body composition and explains the relationship of body composition to performance. Unfortunately, athletes may become obsessed with their weight or body composition. This can lead to overly restricting food intake or exercising to excess. In some cases athletes develop eating disorders, such as anorexia or bulimia, which put their training, performance, and health at risk. These issues are addressed in chapter 11.

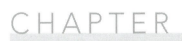

CHAPTER

3

Energy Balance and Imbalance

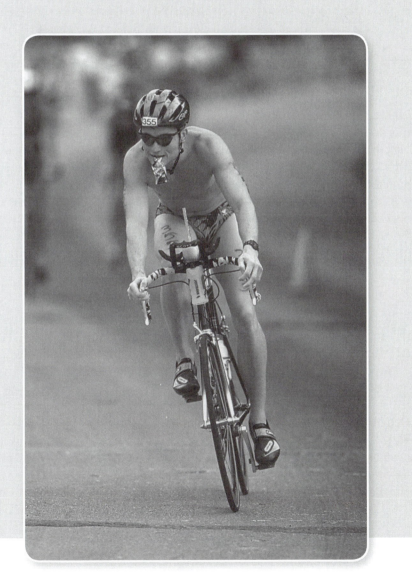

In this chapter, you will learn the following:

✓ Facts about energy and calories

✓ The concepts of "energy in" and "energy out"

✓ Measurement of metabolic rate

✓ Why resistance training and starvation diets influence metabolic rate in very different ways

✓ How a proper diet can help athletes to lose weight without interfering with training or recovery

"Sometimes your body is smarter than you are."

Author unknown

Imagine making it to the top of your sport, only to be hampered by excess body fat. Shaquille O'Neal was nearly 370 pounds (168 kg) in his final season with the Lakers when he was traded to Miami, where he eventually reduced his weight. Jerry Buss, owner of the Lakers, said, "I suspect if I knew he was going to lose 60 pounds (27 kg), I might have made a different decision." Shawn Kemp, an all-star player whose weight had increased to above 300 pounds (136 kg), was cautioned by his general manager, "Until he loses the weight, we don't care if he can score 30 points a game." Kobe Bryant, an NBA star since being drafted out of high school, lost almost 20 pounds (9 kg) after his 10th season in an effort to stay on top of his game. Maintaining body weight is difficult, even for athletes in high-energy-expenditure sports, and excess body fat negatively affects the careers of many athletes, including professionals.

What Is Energy?

Energy is defined as the ability to do work. The energy source that is common to all cells in the body is ATP—adenosine triphosphate. ATP is the direct source of energy for the contraction and relaxation of muscle.

ATP is a compound containing three phosphate groups. When a phosphate group is removed, energy is released. The compound then has two phosphate groups and is known as ADP—adenosine diphosphate. ADP needs to have a phosphate group added in order to form ATP. This process requires an input of energy. The energy needed to resynthesize ATP comes from food.

Figure 3.1 illustrates the big picture. One way to look at energy is to understand that eating food supplies the energy that ADP needs to re-form ATP, which provides the energy for cells to do work. Another way to look at energy is to think about the smallest unit that provides cellular energy, ATP. Energy is released from ATP, resulting in ADP, and something needs to supply the energy to re-form the ATP. That something is food. No matter how you look at it, food and ATP are the bookends.

Food ⟶ ⟶ ⟶ ADP + P ⟶ ATP ⟶ Cellular work

FIGURE 3.1   The big energy picture.

Three Energy Systems

The body has three major energy systems that replenish ATP: creatine phosphate, anaerobic glycolysis, and oxidative phosphorylation, as shown in figure 3.2. The predominant energy system used is determined by the body's need for **speed** and **duration** of ATP replenishment (see table 3.1). In other words, the primary energy system that is used is determined by how quickly ATP is needed and for how long. Creatine phosphate can restore ATP very rapidly but for only a few seconds. It is predominantly used during very high-intensity activities of very short duration. Examples include short sprints such as a 100-meter run, a powerful burst of activity such as a fast break in basketball, or the lifting of a maximal weight such as performing a clean and jerk.

speed—How fast.

duration—How long.

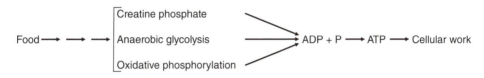

FIGURE 3.2 **The three predominant energy systems (ADP = adenosine diphosphate; P = inorganic phosphate; ATP = adenosine triphosphate).**

Anaerobic glycolysis uses carbohydrate in the absence of oxygen to resynthesize ATP. It is relatively fast but of short duration, about one to two minutes. It is predominantly used during high-intensity, short-duration activities or intermittent activities. Examples include longer sprints such as a 400-meter run, stop-and-go sprints such as in basketball or soccer, and a 15-repetition weightlifting set.

Oxidative phosphorylation, which is also known as the **aerobic** energy system, is the predominant energy system used in many sports. This system is slow compared to the other two systems, but its virtually unlimited replenishment of ATP makes it an ideal energy system when exercise lasts more than a few minutes. Examples include distance running and walking a golf course. This system is also the predominant energy system at rest, such as when sitting or sleeping.

aerobic—In the presence of oxygen.

An analogy is to compare the three energy systems to the first three gears of a manual transmission in a car. First gear is the creatine phosphate system. It gets

TABLE 3.1 Energy Systems Compared

System	Speed	Duration
Creatine phosphate	Very fast	Very short (5-10 seconds)
Anaerobic glycolysis	Fast	Short (1-2 minutes)
Oxidative phosphorylation	Slow	Very long (minutes to many hours)

you off the line in a rush, but it is not long until you have to shift up. Second gear is the anaerobic energy system. It gets you up to speed, but it lasts only a minute or so before you need to shift into third gear. Once in third gear, you can drive for a long time. Similarly, the oxidative phosphorylation system can provide a continuous supply of ATP for activities that last for hours.

carbohydrate—Sugars and starches.

Food is converted into energy in the body. Three sources of energy in food are **carbohydrate**, fat, and protein. As shown in figure 3.3, only carbohydrate can be used for anaerobic glycolysis. All three can be used as a source of energy for the aerobic energy system, oxidative phosphorylation. In this figure, carbohydrate and fat appear in bold because they are the preferred sources of fuel. Alcohol cannot be used directly by muscle cells, so it is not included in figure 3.3.

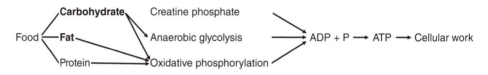

FIGURE 3.3   **How food becomes energy (ADP = adenosine diphosphate; P = inorganic phosphate; ATP = adenosine triphosphate).**

CREATINE PHOSPHATE AND CREATINE

Creatine phosphate (CrP) is a compound that when broken down provides the phosphate and the energy needed to re-form ATP rapidly. Creatine phosphate is predominantly stored in muscle and is broken down in a very rapid, one-step reaction. This makes creatine phosphate an ideal source of energy for very high-intensity activities that last for seconds. However, creatine phosphate in muscle is depleted very rapidly, which is associated with muscle fatigue.

Creatine phosphate is made in the body from creatine and phosphate. The creatine can be supplied in three ways—manufactured in the body, consumed in the diet from beef or fish, or taken as a supplement (see figure 3.4). If no creatine is consumed, the liver and the kidneys make about 2 grams daily from three amino acids easily supplied from dietary protein. Those who eat fish and beef typically consume 1 to 2 grams of creatine per day. These amounts result in a normal creatine level in muscle cells.

Those who supplement typically take 3 to 5 grams of creatine daily. To jump-start the process, first-time users may use a loading dose of 20 to 25 grams daily for the first week

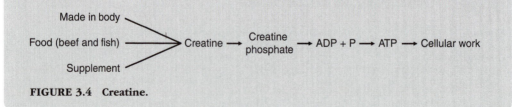

FIGURE 3.4   Creatine.

before reducing intake to a maintenance dose of 3 to 5 grams per day. It is recommended that those who supplement with creatine also consume an adequate amount of fluid.

Studies of athletes in very high-intensity sports, such as sprinters, show a benefit from having maximal levels of creatine phosphate in muscles because CrP is depleted rapidly. Studies also report that supplemental creatine can increase CrP stores in muscle cells by about 20 percent in some people. The largest increases are usually seen in vegetarians. Beef and fish eaters often experience smaller increases because they are already getting creatine from food (Volek & Rawson, 2004).

Maximal CrP levels do not immediately increase strength, power, or speed. However, they may give the athlete the ability to train harder, which can result in improved strength, power, and speed. For example, a sprinter who supplements with creatine may be able to perform more repetitions when weightlifting. More repetitions may increase muscle size and strength, which in turn can improve the sprinter's training (e.g., more sprint repetitions). Scientists refer to this as an indirect performance benefit because the creatine supplement does not directly affect performance. However, the supplementation may allow the sprinter to train harder, longer, or at higher intensity and those factors can improve performance. Athletes in power sports, such as football, hockey, and wrestling frequently use creatine supplements to indirectly improve performance. Bodybuilders are also frequent creatine supplement users in an effort to build maximum muscle mass (Volek & Rawson, 2004).

Studies have shown a direct performance benefit of creatine supplementation for only one sport—powerlifting (Volek & Rawson, 2004). Not surprisingly, creatine supplementation is routine among powerlifters.

Creatine supplementation has been well studied, and there is no evidence that creatine supplements cause dehydration, muscle cramps, or kidney damage. However, it is recommended that those who supplement with creatine also consume an adequate amount of fluid. Supplement use should always be monitored for adverse reactions, such as gastrointestinal upset (GI). Many athletes avoid creatine supplements prior to working out to avoid GI distress. Creatine supplements do increase the amount of water in muscle cells, and wrestlers must account for any increase in water weight due to supplementation or they could be overweight for their desired weight class.

Measuring Energy

In nutrition and exercise physiology, the unit of measurement for energy is the calorie. However, the calorie is too small of a measurement to be useful. It would be like stating your weight in ounces. It is also an outdated term. Therefore, when referring to the measurement of energy in food, this book uses the preferred terms *Calorie* (with a capital *C*) and *kilocalorie*. In the United States the word *calories* (lowercase *c*) is still used as a measurement, although this usage is scientifically incorrect.

For example, 1 tablespoon of oil has 126 Calories, which is abbreviated C or Cal. Calorie is the unit of measurement you will see on food labels in the United States. It is also correct to say that the oil has 126 kilocalories, which is abbreviated kcal and pronounced "k cal." You will likely see this measurement used in technical writing. In articles written for consumers it will probably be written as 126 calories

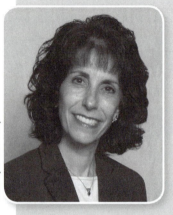
(cal). Technically, the oil has 126,000 calories, which is the equivalent of 126 C or 126 kcal. The terms may be a bit confusing, but regardless of which measurement is used, remember that the caloric content of a food is its energy content.

What Is Energy Balance?

Energy balance occurs when "energy in" equals "energy out," as shown in figure 3.5. The only factor that accounts for "energy in" is the carbohydrate, protein, fat, and alcohol found in food and beverages. Energy is expended in three ways, through **metabolism**, physical activity, and the digestion and use of food. The body cannot create energy or lose energy; it can only transform energy. Thus, the energy contained in food is transformed to biological energy, ATP. If the amount of

metabolism—All the physical and chemical changes that take place in the cells of the body.

energy consumed is equal to the amount of energy expended, then the body is in energy balance.

The body is in energy balance when its percentage of body fat remains stable. Scale weight is highly affected by an athlete's hydration status, which makes it a less desirable choice for assessing energy balance. Energy balance can also be estimated by keeping food and activity diaries and comparing the calories consumed in food and the calories expended by activity, metabolism, and digestion over a period of days or weeks.

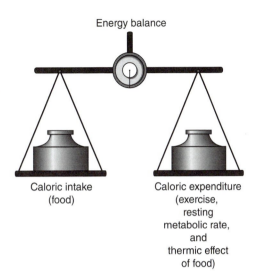

FIGURE 3.5 Energy balance.

Energy In

The energy content of a food depends on the amount of carbohydrate, protein, fat, and alcohol found in that food. Water does not contain any calories. Carbohydrate and protein each contain 4 kilocalories per gram (4 kcal/g), whereas fat contains 9 kcal/g. The approximate caloric content of alcohol is 7 kcal/g. Examples of foods that are essentially pure carbohydrate, protein, fat, or alcohol are listed in table 3.2.

TABLE 3.2   Caloric (Energy) Content of Some Common Foods

Energy-containing component	Food	Weight* (g)	kcal/g	Caloric (energy) content
Carbohydrate	1 sugar cube	4	4 kcal/g	16 kcal
Protein	1 large egg white	4	4 kcal/g	16 kcal
Fat	1 tbsp vegetable oil	14	9 kcal/g	126 kcal
Alcohol (ethanol)	1 shot (1.5 oz) of 80-proof gin, rum, vodka, or whiskey	14	7 kcal/g	98 kcal

g = gram; kcal = kilocalorie; oz = ounce

*Excludes the weight of any water

Many foods are a mixture of various amounts of carbohydrate, protein, or fat. The approximate caloric content is listed either on the label or in an online database such as the one at www.mypyramid.gov. It should be noted that the caloric values are just estimates.

To estimate daily energy intake, athletes can record their food and beverage consumption for 24 hours and enter this information into diet analysis program (page 30). For a more accurate estimate, a food diary should be kept for three to seven days during various training periods, such as the preseason, competitive season, and off-season. Recording food and beverage intake over several days during various training periods helps to better predict energy intake because athletes tend to have variations in their day-to-day, week-to-week, and seasonal caloric intakes.

Studies have shown that a major problem affecting the accuracy of "energy in" estimates is the underreporting of food consumption. This is true for male and female athletes as well as nonathletes. Food intake, and therefore energy intake, is typically underestimated by 10 to 20 percent. In other words, an athlete may estimate his intake to be 3,000 kcal daily, but his actual intake is probably closer to 3,300 to 3,600 kcal. Part of the problem is that people tend to underestimate portion sizes (Magkos & Yannakoulia, 2003).

DIET AND ACTIVITY ANALYSIS PROGRAMS

Computerized programs are available to help people estimate the amount of energy they consume and expend. Some programs are free, but their databases may be limited or the site may be slow as a result of heavy traffic. Programs available for purchase are often comprehensive and allow users to add specialty foods and recipes to the database, but both the initial programs and updates cost money.

Following are some free programs:

MyPyramid.gov: www.mypyramid.gov (click on MyPyramid Tracker)

Shape Up America!: www.shapeup.org (click on Resource Center)

NAT version 2.0: www.nat.uiuc.edu/

Following are programs that are available for purchase:

Food Processor: www.esha.com

Foodworks: www.nutritionco.com

Energy Out

Energy expenditure ("energy out") can be estimated in a manner similar to estimating energy intake and is usually completed at the same time. To estimate daily energy expenditure, record all activities for each 24-hour period, including sleep. This information is then entered into a diet analysis or activity program (see the sidebar above). These programs automatically account for the other components of "energy out"—metabolic rate and the digestion of food.

Studies have shown that the accuracy of activity diaries varies depending on the amount of physical activity performed. Those who have low levels of physical activity tend to overestimate the amount or intensity of the exercise they do. In contrast, those who engage in a high level of activity, such as athletic training and conditioning, tend to underestimate the amount of activity performed, which results in an underestimate of the amount of energy expended (Leenders, Sherman, & Nagaraja, 2006).

A major influence on the "energy out" side of the equation is the degree to which a person is physically active. Sedentary people can achieve energy balance with a relatively low intake of food daily. Athletes in training need substantially more food to provide the calories needed to balance their high energy outputs.

Calories Needed for Energy Balance

The number of calories an athlete needs daily in order to maintain energy balance and current body composition depends to a large degree on the amount of physical activity performed. Although it is more precise to determine each athlete's energy expenditure as described previously, ballpark figures provide a reasonable estimate (see table 3.3).

TABLE 3.3   Estimated Daily Caloric Needs for Male and Female Athletes

Activity level	Examples of activity level	Examples of athletes	Estimated daily caloric need (kcal/kg)	
			Females	**Males**
Sedentary (little physical activity)	Sitting or standing with little activity, for example, desk or computer work, light housekeeping, TV, video games, and so on	During recovery from injury	30	31
Moderate-intensity exercise 3-5 days/week or low-intensity and short-duration training daily	Playing recreational tennis (singles) 1-1 1/2 hr every other day Practicing baseball, softball, or golf 2 1/2 hr daily, 5 days/week	Baseball players Softball players Golfers Recreational tennis players	35	38
Training several hours daily, 5 days/week	Swimming 6,000-10,000 m/day plus some resistance training Doing conditioning and skills training for 2-3 hr/day	Swimmers Soccer players	37	41
Rigorous training on a near daily basis	Performing resistance exercise for 10 to 15 hr/week to maintain well-developed muscle mass Swimming 7,000-17,000 m/day and resistance training 3 days/week	Bodybuilders (maintenance phase) College and professional basketball and American football players Elite swimmers Rugby players	38-40	45
	Training for a triathlon	Non-elite triathletes	41	51.5
Extremely rigorous training	Running 15 mi (24 km)/day or the equivalent	Elite runners, distance cyclists, or triathletes	50 or more	60 or more

kcal/kg = kilocalorie per kilogram of body weight; hr = hour; m = meter; mi = mile; km = kilometer

Reprinted, with permission, from M. Macedonio and M. Dunford, 2009, *Athlete's guide to making weight* (Champaign, IL: Human Kinetics), 82.

These estimates are based on surveys of caloric intakes of athletes at various levels of training and are only approximations. To calculate your daily caloric needs using table 3.3, first determine your weight in kilograms by dividing your weight in pounds by 2.2. Then multiply your weight in kilograms by the number in the column (based on sex) that best describes your activity level. For example, a 130-pound female weighs 59 kg. If she is training several hours daily for five days each week, her estimated daily requirement for maintaining her body weight is about 2,180 kcal (59 kg $\times$ 37 kcal/kg = 2,183 kcal).

Effect of Metabolic Rate on Energy Balance

Sometimes it is beneficial to examine the individual components of energy expenditure such as metabolic rate. Metabolic rate can be used as a guideline to avoid adopting a starvation diet.

Basal metabolic rate (BMR) is the amount of energy needed daily to sustain basic functions such as breathing, body temperature, and blood circulation. BMR must be measured under precise laboratory conditions in which the room temperature is controlled and the person lies absolutely still. It is more practical to measure **resting metabolic rate** (RMR). RMR is about 10 percent higher than BMR because precise conditions cannot be duplicated outside of a laboratory.

resting metabolic rate—An estimate of the amount of energy needed to keep the body alive at rest.

Factors that influence metabolic rate include age, sex, genetics, height, and hormones, particularly thyroid hormones. These influences may differentiate people from one another (e.g., "I have a higher metabolic rate than my father"), but they are not under voluntary control so there is little that one can do to influence them.

Some factors such as caffeine intake, cigarette smoking, change in altitude or environmental temperature, and exercise cause a temporary rise in metabolic rate. Most of these factors have a small influence on metabolic rate.

The two factors under voluntary control that have the most influence on metabolic rate are the amount of **fat-free tissue** and severe restriction of food intake. However, these two factors influence metabolic rate in very different ways. Increasing skeletal muscle mass through resistance training is the most logical way to increase metabolic rate. On the other hand, severe caloric restriction decreases metabolic rate. Starvation diets, even for a few days, can reduce metabolic rate by 20 percent or more. Not only does RMR decrease, but it also remains depressed for weeks even after the person begins eating an adequate amount of food.

fat-free tissue—The tissues in the body that are not fat, such as muscle, organs, and bones.

Resting metabolic rate can be measured using a metabolic cart, which is often found in exercise physiology laboratories or training centers for elite athletes. Smaller, portable systems are also available at some fitness centers or health clubs. In many cases athletes do not have access to the equipment needed to measure RMR. Instead, they obtain a ballpark figure by using one of the formulas shown in the sidebar Estimating Resting Metabolic Rate on page 33.

Most athletes use an estimate of RMR to make sure they are not restricting calories too severely when they attempt to lose body fat. For example, the resting metabolic rate of a 220-pound (100 kg) male is estimated to be around 2,400 kcal. Reducing caloric intake to 1,000 kcal even for a couple of days would likely reduce his RMR because he would be starving himself. Severely restricting caloric intake forces the body to conserve energy, and one way it does this is to reduce RMR.

Estimating Resting Metabolic Rate

The most accurate estimate of resting metabolic rate for athletes is the Cunningham equation, but body composition must first be taken to determine fat-free mass (Thompson & Manore, 1996). The least accurate but easiest method is to use the simplified formula.

CUNNINGHAM EQUATION

RMR = 500 + 22 (FFM in kg)

SIMPLIFIED FORMULA

Men: 1 kcal/kg body weight/hr × 24 hr
  Example: 1 kcal × 75 kg × 24 hr = 1,800 kcal

Women: 0.9 kcal/kg body weight/hr × 24 hr
  Example: 0.9 kcal × 75 kg × 24 hr = 1,620 kcal

FFM = fat-free mass; kg = kilogram; kcal = kilocalorie; hr = hour

Effect of TEF on Energy Balance

After food is consumed, there is a slight increase in energy expenditure as the food is digested, absorbed, and transported to cells. This temporary increase is known as the thermic effect of food (TEF). TEF is estimated to be approximately 10 percent of total caloric intake. For example, a person who consumes 2,500 kcal daily may use as much as 250 kcal to digest, absorb, and use the nutrients contained in that food.

In most cases, TEF is not a concern to athletes because the amount of energy used is small, particularly when compared to the energy expended via metabolic rate and physical activity. However, a few athletes, such as bodybuilders, may be looking for ways to increase energy expenditure in an effort to burn as many calories as possible and attain an extremely low percentage of body fat. Protein has the greatest effect on TEF, followed by carbohydrate; fat has very little effect. Therefore, a bodybuilder may alter his diet to emphasize protein foods and nearly eliminate fat-containing foods. Theoretically, this diet composition would result in a small increase in energy expenditure as a result of a slightly increased TEF. However, in practice, eating a high-protein, high-carbohydrate, very low-fat diet will have only a minor effect on the number of calories the body expends.

What Is Energy Imbalance?

If energy balance is "energy in = energy out," then energy imbalance means that the two sides of the equation are not equal. The most common imbalance in the United States and other Western countries is that energy intake via food is greater than energy expenditure. This results in an accumulation of body fat as the excess calories are stored in **adipose tissue**. Less frequent, but as difficult to change, is a caloric intake that is too low for daily energy expenditure. This imbalance leads to being underweight with marginal fat stores. In such cases the person may lack appetite, which makes increasing food intake unappealing and difficult.

adipose tissue—Body fat stores.

Many athletes want to decrease body fat. Reasons include wanting to improve performance, especially if weight needs to be moved, such as in distance running or high jumping; subjective scoring that favors a relatively low percentage of body fat or thin appearance, such as in women's gymnastics and figure skating; wanting to improve personal appearance; and desiring better health, which is particularly true for recreational athletes. The challenge is to reduce overall caloric intake but not to the point at which metabolic rate is reduced or the amount of nutrients needed to support training, performance, recovery, and health is inadequate.

> *After a couple of years of helping the same athletes achieve the same goal (weight loss), I realized that in order to be successful in sport, athletes needed to have their nutrition support their training. Most athletes know what periodization is and I simply provided the basis of including nutrition into their physical training cycles and body weight/composition goals. Hence, my mantra, "eat to train, don't train to eat" was born!*
>
> Bob Seebohar, MS, RD, CSSD, CSCS, author of *Nutrition Periodization for Endurance Athletes: Taking Traditional Sports Nutrition to the Next Level*

How Can Athletes Reduce Body Fat?

Body fat is reduced when there is a caloric deficit over time. The fundamental principle remains the same regardless of the specific program followed—eat less, exercise more, or do both. As a rule of thumb, 1 pound (0.5 kg) of body fat contains about 3,500 kcal. Mathematically, if a person reduced food intake and increased exercise by a combined 500 kcal daily, then in seven days' time he or she would lose 1 pound of body fat. Such estimates are correct, but a 500 kcal deficit is very difficult to achieve for most sedentary people, many recreational athletes, and many small-bodied athletes whose caloric intake is relatively low. Losing substantial amounts of body fat takes time and sustained motivation.

There is no shortage of advice on the subject of weight loss, but when applied to athletes there are some important issues to consider. The most important are timing, degree of calorie restriction, composition of the diet, and avoiding strategies that will undermine training, recovery, and performance. Athletes need to understand the following:

- Weight loss is not necessarily fat loss.
- Rapid weight loss is usually a result of water and glycogen loss as well as some muscle, which can hamper training, performance, recovery, and health.
- A realistic expectation is the loss of 1 to 2 pounds (0.5 to 1 kg) of body fat per week. A 20-pound (9 kg) loss can take two and a half to five months, so athletes must plan accordingly.
- The best time for most athletes to lose body fat is in the off-season or early in the preseason.
- Restricting calories during periods of rigorous training or competition may hamper training, recovery, or performance.
- Daily caloric intake should be less than usual, but too great a restriction will likely result in too low of a carbohydrate intake to support training and recovery.
- Adequate protein intake and resistance exercise help to offset the loss of muscle during moderate calorie restriction.
- Exercise above usual training levels must be chosen carefully to prevent overuse injuries.

Nutrition Bite

Which weight loss diet is the best—low fat or low carbohydrate?

No debate has been more passionate than the one about what is the best weight loss diet. On one side are the supporters of a low-fat diet who point out that it is easy to overconsume fat and it has more calories per gram than carbohydrate, protein, or alcohol. Others say that a low-carbohydrate diet is best. This type of diet allows people to eat protein and fat-containing foods and eliminates nearly all sugars and most starches. So which type of diet is best?

Scientists studied people on different types of weight loss diets. They discovered that it didn't matter whether the diet was low in fat or low in carbohydrate as long as it was lower in calories. They also discovered that many people had a hard time following any diet (Sacks et al., 2009).

So, which weight loss diet is best? The one the person can stay on!

Unfortunately, many athletes fall prey to the quick fixes and rapid weight loss programs that are so heavily advertised. These programs generally suggest severe calorie restriction so weight loss is rapid. However, it is recommended that athletes consume no less than 30 kcal per kilogram of body weight daily. For example, a 154-pound (70 kg) athlete who wants to lose body fat should not typically consume less than 2,100 kcal daily. This caloric level is above resting metabolic rate and is not considered a starvation-type diet. Caloric restriction below this level will typically not provide enough of the carbohydrate, protein, and fat needed to maintain training or conditioning.

A tool that can help athletes create a personalized fat loss plan is the daily energy intake and expenditure estimates described earlier in this chapter. A good rule of thumb is to create a daily calorie deficit of about 500 kcal. For example, an athlete may look at his usual food intake and activity level and find that he could

Nutrition Bite

Why do starvation diets make things worse? To lose body fat, a person must create a calorie deficit. It may seem logical that the bigger the caloric restriction is, the larger and faster the fat loss will be, but in fact, the larger the caloric restriction is, the more problems are created. Starvation diets make things worse for the following reasons:

- Muscle mass is lost with a starvation diet.
- The body lowers metabolic rate and keeps it lower for weeks after the starvation diet ends.
- Starvation diets are typically followed by weight gain.
- Starvation diets may encourage binge eating and lead to yo-yo dieting, which is a constant cycle of weight loss followed by weight gain.

realistically decrease his food intake by 400 kcal daily and increase his exercise by 100 kcal daily. In some cases, such as with small-bodied athletes, a 500 kcal daily deficit would be too much, but a 200 kcal decrease in intake and a 100 kcal increase in exercise (such as resistance exercise) would be achievable, although fat loss would occur at a slower rate.

Once the athlete has established a daily total caloric intake goal, she must determine the distribution of calories for a weight loss diet. Approximately 1.5 grams of protein per kilogram of body weight, or 20 percent of the total calories, should come from protein to help preserve muscle mass and metabolic rate. For example, the 154-pound (70 kg) athlete would need about 105 grams of protein daily, an amount that is not difficult to obtain from food. The majority of the remaining calories should come from carbohydrate, but it is important that the diet have sufficient fat (~20 to 25 percent of total calories) to satisfy hunger. Generally, alcohol is eliminated from the diet when an athlete is trying to lose body fat.

Athletes may find it beneficial to eat six small meals or snacks daily. If possible, each meal or snack should contain some carbohydrate, protein, and fat to keep blood sugar level stable, to repair and protect muscle, and to keep the athlete from getting too hungry.

To summarize, it is typically recommended that athletes who want to lose body fat do the following:

- Consume no less than 30 kcal per kilogram of body weight daily
- Create a calorie deficit of about 300-500 kcal daily, with some of the deficit resulting from a reduction in food intake and some resulting from an increase in physical activity (adjust as necessary)
- Consume about 1.5 grams of protein per kilogram of body weight daily

- Eat six small meals or snacks daily
- Continue or include resistance training to help preserve muscle mass

How Can Athletes Gain Body Fat?

Although it receives much less attention, an athlete may be underweight with marginal body fat stores, which can have a negative effect on performance, recovery, and health. It is important to determine why the athlete is underweight. Those who are underweight because of disordered eating need specialized medical, nutritional, and psychological counseling (see chapter 11). However, some underweight people eat normally. They are called constitutionally thin.

Limited studies of constitutionally thin women have found that they have been thin all their lives and have family members who are thin, suggesting a genetic predisposition to thinness. Because their daily caloric intake is equal to their energy expenditure, weight and percentage of body fat are stable. Some would like to gain weight, but find it difficult to do so (Bossu et al., 2007).

Based on the energy equation, to gain weight as body fat, a person must consume more calories than she expends. It may seem intuitive that this could easily be accomplished by eating high-fat, high-sugar foods, such as milkshakes. However, such foods are filling and can suppress appetite. One cannot gain weight if a 400 kcal milkshake replaces a 600 kcal meal. Instead, the typical advice is to increase the portion sizes of foods already being consumed and supplement the current diet with heart-healthy fat sources such nuts, seeds, and avocadoes. It may also help to eat more frequently, even if hunger is absent.

> *However beautiful the strategy, you should occasionally look at the results.*
>
> **Winston Churchill**, who served as prime minister
> of the United Kingdom during World War II

The Short of It

- Energy is the ability to do work.
- Energy balance is defined as "energy in = energy out."
- Food is "energy in."
- Foods with carbohydrate and protein have about 4 kcal/g, alcohol has about 7 kcal/g, and fat has about 9 kcal/g.
- Metabolism, activity, and the thermic effect of food are "energy out."
- When "energy in" exceeds "energy out," the body stores the excess energy as body fat.
- Increasing the amount of muscle mass increases metabolic rate.

- Starvation diets decrease metabolic rate and can cause other problems.
- Athletes must plan ahead to allow enough time to lose the desired amount of body fat.
- Athletes wishing to lose weight need a moderately reduced-calorie diet with sufficient protein, carbohydrate, and fat to train and recover properly.

CHAPTER

Carbohydrate

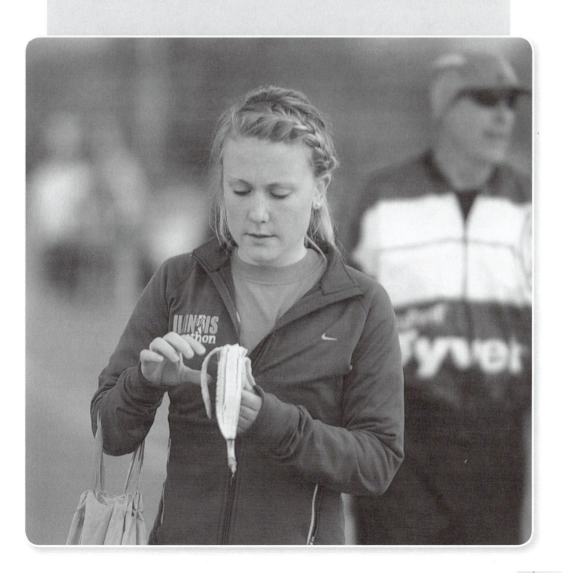

In this chapter, you will learn the following:

✓ Where carbohydrate is found in food and in the body
✓ The importance of carbohydrate for athletic performance
✓ How much carbohydrate is recommended daily for athletes in training
✓ How much carbohydrate should be consumed before, during, and after exercise
✓ Facts about carbohydrate loading

"Why aren't you signed up for the 401K?"

"I'd never be able to run that far."

From the comic strip Dilbert, written by Scott Adams (April 2, 2001)

This is Jared's story:

Over a couple of beers one night, my best friend bet me that I couldn't finish a marathon. Never one to shy away from a bet, I decided to sign up for the Chicago race, which was three months away. My training was sporadic, but I'm a pretty strong runner and I was feeling pretty solid on my occasional 10-mile runs. It was a six-hour drive to Chicago, and we took off later than we had planned so we didn't stop to eat, but we grabbed a few snacks when we filled up for gas. By the time we checked into the hotel, it was almost midnight and we were starved. We settled for dinner at the nearest fast-food restaurant where I told them to supersize it. After all, I was going to run a marathon. The next morning I overslept so there was no time for breakfast.

Everything was going OK until about mile 19 when I began to feel like I was dragging my feet—as if I had exchanged my running shoes for scuba fins. I slowed my pace but kept going and at mile 20 I saw my best buddy cheering me on. His skin looked an odd color of green. About a mile later he showed up again, but this time he was bright blue. At the same time I felt as if another runner had jumped on my back but I was too tired to argue with him and I figured I'd just bring the both of us to the finish line even if we had to crawl there. After about another half mile I noticed that all the other runners were running toward me. Next thing I knew I was looking at the pavement. That's when some guy knelt down and said, "Hey, buddy, I think you're done. The medics are on their way." Later I found out that I had "bonked" because I had run out of glycogen.

What Is Carbohydrate and How Does It Relate to Exercise?

Carbohydrates are compounds that contain carbon, hydrogen, and oxygen (CHO). They are found in food as **sugars**, **starches**, and **fiber**. In the body, carbohydrates are found as glucose and glycogen. Glucose is blood sugar and glycogen is the storage form of carbohydrate found in the muscles and liver.

Carbohydrate is the primary source of fuel for the muscles during moderate to intense exercise. Much of the carbohydrate comes from muscle glycogen. Muscle glycogen is depleted by exercise and is restored by eating a sufficient amount of carbohydrate daily. Consuming enough carbohydrate every day is very important for athletes because those with depleted muscle glycogen stores cannot continue to exercise at the same intensity or for as long.

sugar—A simple form of carbohydrate.

starch—Chains of glucose molecules; also used to describe foods containing many chains of glucose, such as potatoes.

fiber—A type of carbohydrate that cannot be digested.

Exercising muscle prefers to use muscle glycogen if it is available. However, glucose (blood sugar) is also a source of fuel. Glucose is provided to the blood during exercise primarily by the breakdown of liver glycogen or the consumption of carbohydrate foods and beverages. The amount of glucose provided by the breakdown of liver glycogen is relatively small and the process is slow. Carbohydrate foods and beverages consumed during exercise can provide a steady stream of glucose, but there are limits to how much and how fast carbohydrate can be absorbed from the intestinal tract.

Carbohydrate intake is often associated with endurance athletes such as distance runners and cyclists. The demand for carbohydrate during moderate- to high-intensity, long-duration exercise is high, and these athletes run the risk of running out of muscle glycogen before the race is over. Therefore, endurance athletes focus on having sufficient muscle glycogen stores by consuming enough carbohydrate daily to resynthesize the muscle glycogen used during daily training and competition. They also depend on consuming beverages, gels, and foods that contain carbohydrate during endurance exercise.

Nutrition Bite

What happened to Jared, the runner in the opening paragraph of this chapter? Jared made many mistakes that resulted in his not finishing the race. Here are some of the things that went wrong:

- He trained sporadically.
- He ate a high-fat, low-carbohydrate meal the night before the race.
- He ate no food before the race.
- He became disoriented because his blood sugar was low.
- He could no longer continue to exercise because his muscle glycogen was depleted.

Many recreational athletes do not realize the importance of sufficient carbohydrate. Eating a low-carbohydrate meal the night before the race meant that Jared started the race with less than optimal glycogen stores. He didn't add to the stores in the morning because he did not eat before the competition. If he had had a better eating plan, he might have been able to finish the race and not lose the bet with his buddy!

But long-duration athletes are not the only ones who need adequate muscle glycogen stores. Carbohydrate is also the predominant source of energy for high-intensity, short-duration exercise lasting about one or two minutes. Soccer and basketball are examples of sports in which players repeatedly sprint for short periods of time. These are referred to as stop-and-go sports, and these athletes also need sufficient glycogen stores. Both endurance and stop-and-go athletes can deplete muscle glycogen stores during training and competition.

Some athletes deplete muscle glycogen during training but not competition. For example, a swimmer who repeatedly swims 50- to 100-meter intervals can deplete muscle glycogen during training. Similarly, the athlete who is doing 10 to 15 repetitions for each of 15 sets during weight training uses some muscle glycogen. Muscle glycogen needs to be restored before the next training session. However, a 100-meter swim during competition is not long enough to deplete muscle glycogen.

Many athletes engage in rigorous training programs that deplete muscle glycogen on a near-daily basis. Thus, most athletes need to be concerned about their daily intake of carbohydrate foods so they can replenish depleted glycogen stores each day. Athletes competing in long-duration events or in bodybuilding competitions strive to have maximum muscle glycogen stores before competition. They increase their carbohydrate intake and reduce the amount of exercise a few days before the competitive event to ensure that they begin the competition with as much muscle glycogen as possible. This procedure is known as carbohydrate loading and is explained later in this chapter.

> *Essentially, we distinguish ourselves from the rest. If you want to win something, run the 100 meters. If you want to experience something, run a marathon.*
>
> **Emil Zátopek**, winner of three gold medals in the 1952 summer Olympics—5K, 10K, and the marathon, which he entered at the last minute and was the first marathon he had ever run

What Are the Daily Carbohydrate Recommendations?

All athletes should consume at least 5 grams of carbohydrate per kilogram of body weight per day (5 g/kg/d) or at least 50 percent of total calories as carbohydrate. For example, a 150-pound (68 kg) person should consume at least 340 grams of carbohydrate daily (68 kg × 5 g/kg = 340 g). A sample menu containing this amount of carbohydrate is shown on page 43. Consuming less carbohydrate will likely result in low muscle glycogen stores.

However, many athletes need more than the minimum amount of carbohydrate because they need to replenish the large amount of muscle glycogen depleted with rigorous daily training. It is generally recommended that athletes who are rigorously training, such as college American football players, consume up to 7 g/kg

SAMPLE DAILY MENU CONTAINING APPROXIMATELY 340 GRAMS OF CARBOHYDRATE

Breakfast

1 cup orange juice

1 cup cooked oatmeal

1 teaspoon margarine

1 medium banana

1 cup nonfat milk

Lunch

2 slices wheat bread

4 ounces (125 g) lean turkey

2 teaspoons mustard

15 baked potato chips

1 medium orange

1/4 cup trail mix (fruit and nuts)

Snack

12 ounces (360 ml) sport drink

2 large graham cracker squares

Dinner

1 1/2 cup spaghetti noodles

1 cup spaghetti sauce

1 cup cooked carrots

1 medium slice French bread

2 teaspoons margarine

Snack

8 ounces (240 ml) low-fat chocolate milk

Total carbohydrate from this menu is 344 grams or 5 g/kg (grams of carbohydrate per kilogram of body weight) or 63 percent of total calories. This is based on a 150-pound (68 kg) athlete.

daily. This amount of dietary carbohydrate restores muscle glycogen to a level that allows athletes to train hard on consecutive days. However, this is a moderately high amount (approximately 70 percent of total calories), and many athletes find it hard to consume this much carbohydrate.

Highly trained endurance and stop-and-go athletes typically need more than 7 g/kg of carbohydrate daily to fully replenish the muscle glycogen depleted during rigorous in-season training and competition. It is recommended that such athletes consume 8 to 10 g/kg/d so that muscle glycogen levels are fully replenished each day and remain high over the months of rigorous training. This is a large amount of carbohydrate daily (about 80 percent of total calories), and it is often difficult for athletes to stay within this range or reach the top end of the range. Near-maximum muscle glycogen stores are recommended before competition; otherwise, the athlete is at risk of running low on muscle glycogen during the event. Muscle glycogen depletion is known as hitting the wall or bonking and results in early fatigue or an inability to finish the competition, as was the case of Jared in this chapter's opening story.

Ultraendurance athletes, such as triathletes and Tour de France riders, are covering such long distances that their carbohydrate needs are tremendously high. The goal for carbohydrate intake for ultraendurance athletes during competition or heavy training periods may be above 10 g/kg/d. Such a large intake requires frequent carbohydrate feedings before, during,

Ultraendurance—Very prolonged endurance activities. *Ultra* means "excessive."

Nutrition Bite

"Shh!" whispered one wrestler to another, "I'm on a low-carbohydrate diet and I don't want coach to know. I need to lose weight fast so I'm going to follow the Atkins' diet for just a couple of weeks."

The Atkins' diet restricts carbohydrate intake to 20 grams per day for the first 14 days and approximately 20 to 60 grams per day after the first two weeks. For many people, this would be the equivalent of 5 to 15 percent of total calories as carbohydrates. Such a low-carbohydrate intake by an athlete is disadvantageous because muscle glycogen stores would be too low, making it difficult to train.

Why would an athlete even think about consuming a low-carbohydrate diet? Because studies have shown that in the short term (around 12 weeks), low-carbohydrate diets are more effective than low-fat diets in reducing weight and body fat. However, the advantages associated with rapid weight loss will likely be offset by the disadvantages associated with not being able to train as long or as hard.

and after training as well as frequent meals and snacks whenever they are awake (Seebohar, 2006).

Surveys suggest that many athletes fall short of the recommended intake of carbohydrate, as shown in table 4.1. In some cases this is due to taking in too little food overall. In other words, these athletes are restricting their calorie intake, often in an effort to lose body fat, so their carbohydrate intake is low, too. However, some athletes are consuming an adequate number of calories but they are eating foods that are high in protein and fat. These athletes are also not consuming a sufficient amount of carbohydrate.

Daily carbohydrate intake is emphasized because of the consequences of low muscle glycogen stores. In the early 1970s, Costill and colleagues (1971) studied well-trained distance runners and found that a moderate carbohydrate diet (around 5 g/kg) failed to restore muscle glycogen levels after a 10-mile (16 km) run. When studied on successive days, muscle glycogen stores declined in a stepwise fashion,

TABLE 4.1 Usual Versus Recommended Carbohydrate Intake by Athletes

	Average CHO intake (g/kg/d)	Recommended CHO intake (g/kg/d)
Female, nonendurance	4.6	5-7
Male, nonendurance	5.8	5-7
Female, endurance	5.7	7-10
Male, endurance	7.6	7-10

CHO= carbohydrate; g = gram; kg = kilograms of body weight; d= day

Data from Burke, Kiens, & Ivy, 2004.

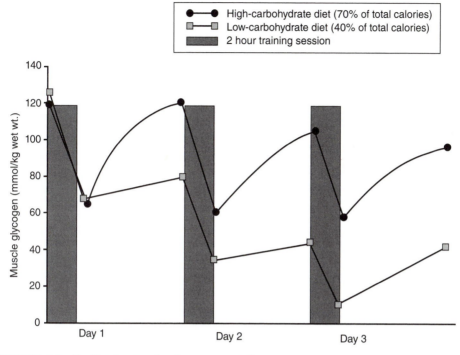

FIGURE 4.1   Decline in muscle glycogen over time.

Adapted from D.L. Costill et al., 1971, "Muscle glycogen utilization during prolonged exercise on successive days," *Journal of Applied Physiology* 31: 836. Used with permission.

as shown in figure 4.1. As documented in other studies, the gradual reduction in muscle glycogen stores leads to an inability to continue training and has a negative impact on performance.

Sources of Carbohydrate

Carbohydrate is found in foods as sugar, starch, and fiber. Sugars found naturally in foods include fructose (fruit sugar) and lactose (milk sugar). Sugars such as sucrose (white, or table, sugar) are also added to foods. **High-fructose corn syrup** is frequently used to sweeten drinks, such as soft drinks.

Starches are long chains of glucose and are abundant in grains such as wheat, rice, and oats, and in products made from grains, such as bread, cereal, pastas, and tortillas. Other examples of starches are beans, such as soy and pinto beans, and starchy vegetables, such as potatoes and yams. Enzymes

high-fructose corn syrup—A syrup made by combining corn syrup, which is nearly 100 percent glucose, and fructose.

in the intestinal tract break down starches to glucose, which can then be absorbed. In contrast, the human intestinal tract is not capable of breaking fiber down because it lacks the enzymes to do so. Despite the inability to be absorbed, dietary fiber is necessary for good health because it maintains bowel function and lowers the risk of getting heart disease and diabetes.

Sugars and starches both contain 4 kcal/g. Thus, 30 grams of sugar and 30 grams of starch have the same caloric content—120 kcal. However, there are important differences in their nutrient contents. Minimally processed carbohydrate foods, such as whole-grain breads and cereals, dried beans and legumes, nuts, vegetables, and fruits contain many vitamins, minerals, and fiber. On the other hand, white sugar lacks fiber, vitamins, and minerals. Unfortunately, most grain products in grocery stores today are not made from minimally processed whole grains. Instead, the grains are highly processed, which removes the fiber, and sweetened with sugar, which adds calories without adding nutrients.

This has led to carbohydrates being labeled good or bad. Whole-grain, nutrient-rich foods are often referred to as good, whereas highly processed, high-sugar

⭐ SUCCESS STORY

Ellen Coleman, The Sport Clinic

Ellen Coleman, MA, MPH, RD, CSSD, learned an important lesson about the exercise physiology lab as a master's student at the University of California at Davis: Never come in late or you will be the one chosen to participate in the next experiment that requires a rectal temperature! There were many other things she learned, among them the importance of carbohydrate in endurance performance. Ellen's knowledge of carbohydrate extends well beyond the classroom because she is an endurance athlete herself and twice finished the Hawaii Ironman triathlon.

Ellen has been one of the most respected sport dietitians since the field emerged in the early 1980s. She is the nutrition consultant for The Sport Clinic in Riverside, California, and has advised many of the professional teams in the Los Angeles area. She was one of the first to write a book about diet and performance, aptly named *Eating for Endurance*. In addition, she has written a nutrition column for *Sports Medicine Digest* for more

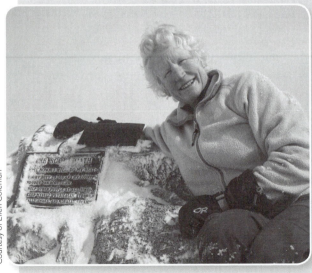

than 20 years and has conducted numerous continuing education courses for professionals.

Not only is Ellen a recognized authority on sport nutrition, but she also tries to combat nutrition quackery. She has received numerous awards for achievement and excellence in practice. One of her catch phrases is "miles of smiles," something athletes will experience if they follow her advice about diet and athletic performance. Her personal and professional achievements have set a high standard for anyone who is considering a career in sport nutrition.

Courtesy of Ellen Coleman

foods are deemed bad. The problem with such categorizations is that there is no accounting for the situation in which the foods are consumed. Highly processed, highly sugared foods are very appropriate for athletes during and immediately after exercise because of their rapid absorption and low fiber content. Nutrient content is a low priority for the athlete at that time. This is a classic example of how what is considered a bad food is actually good under the right circumstance. That said, many athletes consume too many highly processed, high-sugar, low-nutrient foods and beverages throughout the day and need to eat more whole grains, dried beans, and vegetables.

Carbohydrate-Rich Foods

Certain food groups contain substantial amounts of carbohydrate making it easier for athletes to plan a carbohydrate-rich diet that is also nutrient-rich. Fruits, vegetables, grains, beans, milk, and nuts are all food groups that contribute carbohydrate as well as other nutrients. Foods are grouped together because they contain a similar amount of carbohydrate, but there are differences in nutrient content among the foods in each group. For example, iceberg lettuce and spinach are both vegetables, but spinach has more nutrients than iceberg lettuce has.

Fruits   One serving of a fruit typically contains between 10 and 20 grams of carbohydrate. A serving is usually defined as a small piece of fruit about 2 1/2 inches (6.4 cm) in diameter or 1/2 cup of fruit juice. Fruits such as oranges and strawberries are excellent sources of vitamin C, and cantaloupes, mangoes, and papayas provide substantial amounts of vitamin A. Apples, bananas, and blueberries are good sources of fiber, although most fruits provide some fiber.

Vegetables   *Vegetable* is a term that is sometimes used to describe both starchy and nonstarchy vegetables, which vary considerably in their carbohydrate and nutrient contents. One-half cup of a starchy vegetable, such as corn, potatoes, and yams, contains about 15 grams of carbohydrate per serving.

A half-cup serving of orange or green, leafy vegetables such as carrots, winter squash, tomatoes, or broccoli contains about 5 grams of carbohydrate. These vegetables are also excellent sources of vitamin A, and some, such as cabbage, broccoli, tomatoes, and peppers, provide vitamin C. Most vegetables are also good sources of fiber.

Experts recommend that adults consume at least five servings of fruits and vegetables daily. Athletes are generally encouraged to consume more. Consuming a variety of fruits and vegetables each day is strongly recommended because they vary in nutrient content.

Grains   Grains often contain between 15 and 45 grams of carbohydrate depending on the portion size, so they are sometimes grouped in 15-gram increments. One-half cup of a cooked cereal grain, such as oatmeal, 1/3 cup cooked rice or pasta, or 1 slice of bread contains about 15 grams of carbohydrate. One ounce of chips, such as potato chips or corn chips, also has 15 grams, but chips contain more sodium and fat than the aforementioned products do.

A 1-cup portion of ready-to-eat (cold) cereal has about 30 grams of carbohydrate, as do many granola bars. Three 4-inch (10 cm) pancakes and one 10-inch (25 cm) flour tortilla also provide 30 grams of carbohydrate each. Unless these products are made from whole grains, they typically do not provide a substantial amount of fiber, although each product does have some. Because portion sizes have gotten bigger over the past two decades, many grain products today have 30 to 45 grams of carbohydrate per serving. Examples include 4- to 5-inch (10 to 13 cm) bagels, energy bars, and large, soft pretzels.

Adults should consume at least three servings of whole grains daily for good health. Athletes often obtain a substantial amount of their daily carbohydrate from the grain group.

Sweetened grain is a term for a grain product that has a substantial amount of sugar added. In many cases fat and sodium have been added, too. A bowl of oatmeal is a whole grain, but an oatmeal cookie is a sweetened grain. The best way to find out more information about grain products in the United States is to read the food label, Nutrition Facts. The label will state the grams of total carbohydrate, dietary fiber, and sugars in one serving of the product. Information is also provided about calories, fat, cholesterol, sodium, protein, and several vitamins and minerals.

Beans   Beans and legumes provide about 20 grams of carbohydrate per half-cup serving of cooked beans. Nearly every region of the world has traditional bean dishes—soybeans (Asia), garbanzo beans (Middle east), split peas (Scandinavia), navy beans (Eastern United States), black beans (South America), and pinto beans (Southwestern United States and Mexico). Beans contain a substantial amount of fiber and also contribute some protein to the diet. Canned beans often form the basis of a quick meal for athletes because they do not have to be refrigerated, can be cooked quickly, and are relatively inexpensive.

Milk   One cup (8 oz or 240 ml) of milk contains about 12 grams of carbohydrate; chocolate milk has twice that amount. One cup of plain yogurt or soy milk typically has at least 17 grams, but flavored yogurt can have more if sugar has been added. This food group provides a substantial amount of calcium, but many people cannot tolerate dairy products because they are **lactose intolerant**.

lactose intolerant—Unable to fully digest lactose (milk sugar), resulting in gastrointestinal upset.

Nuts   Nuts and seeds are sometimes overlooked as a source of carbohydrate and fiber because of their fat content. Two tablespoons of peanut butter contains 6 grams of carbohydrate along with 16 grams of heart-healthy fat and 190 kcal. This may be advantageous for an athlete who expends a lot of calories daily and needs a concentrated source of energy that is easy and available. However, many athletes would easily exceed their caloric goal for the day if they included too large a portion of nuts.

Sugar   Some common sources of sugar are white sugar, honey, maple syrup, high-fructose corn syrup, brown sugar, jams and jellies, and sugar-sweetened beverages including sport beverages. One teaspoon of sugar contains 4 grams of carbohydrate. Most 12-ounce (360 ml) soft drinks contain about 8 teaspoons of sugar. Sugar is added to many foods because people like sweet-tasting foods. For example, 1 tablespoon of ketchup contains 1 teaspoon of sugar.

Carbohydrate Products Developed Specifically for Athletes

Many carbohydrate-containing products have been developed specifically for athletes making it easier to obtain the amount and type of carbohydrate needed. For example, sport beverages were first developed in 1965 to help meet the fluid, carbohydrate, and electrolyte needs of athletes competing in the heat. They are formulated to provide about 15 grams per 8-ounce (240 ml) serving. The concentration of carbohydrate is typically 6 to 8 percent, which aids rapid absorption and lowers the risk of gastrointestinal distress.

The sport beverage product line has been expanded to meet the specific needs of athletes, particularly endurance athletes. For example, some beverages contain glucose polymers—chains of glucose—that are slowly absorbed and provide a steady stream of glucose into the blood over time. Recovery beverages provide more carbohydrate than those consumed during exercise. These beverages contain some sugars that are absorbed quickly for the purpose of restoring muscle glycogen rapidly.

Carbohydrate products other than beverages have been developed, especially for endurance and ultraendurance athletes. Sport gels provide 25 grams of carbohydrate per packet. These gels are easy to open and consume during exercise. Sport bars with an equivalent amount of carbohydrate are also available because athletes who exercise continuously for hours often like some "solid" food, along with gels and beverages. Recovery bars provide some rapidly absorbed carbohydrate, usually from a variety of sugars.

Athletes should evaluate the content of any product and test it during training. They should read the ingredient label to determine what is in the product (e.g., grams of carbohydrate) and whether the product is appropriate for the situation. It cannot be emphasized enough that athletes should test during training any product they plan to consume before or during competition to determine their **gastrointestinal** tolerance. It may be tempting for a marathon runner to try a new beverage, gel, or bar that is available along the course, but trying a new product for the first time during competition is not recommended.

> **gastrointestinal**—Relating to the stomach and the intestines.

Distribution of Daily Carbohydrate Intake

The total amount of carbohydrate to be consumed daily is one concern, but how that carbohydrate is distributed across the day is important, too. Guidelines have been developed for carbohydrate intake before, during, and after exercise. The amount and timing of carbohydrate intake depends on the intensity and duration of the exercise as well as the athlete's gastrointestinal tolerances.

Before Exercise

Athletes' choices of carbohydrate foods and drinks to consume in the hours before exercise are based on specific goals. A goal for all athletes is to minimize gastrointestinal distress (nausea, vomiting, abdominal cramping, or diarrhea). Other goals may be to prevent hunger, stabilize blood sugar, or top off muscle glycogen stores to delay fatigue during exercise. Being adequately hydrated before exercise is also a goal, and athletes often choose carbohydrate-containing beverages to kill two birds with one stone.

The first step in knowing how much carbohydrate to consume before exercise is to determine how much time one has before exercise begins. During exercise the flow of blood to the muscles increases and the blood flow to the gastrointestinal tract decreases. This means that digestion is likely to be delayed. Too much of a food or beverage too close to the time of exercise may result in gastrointestinal distress such as nausea, bloating, or intestinal cramps.

As a rule of thumb, a meal can be comfortably consumed three or four hours before exercise. Meals can meet all the athlete's preexercise goals by satisfying hunger, providing some glucose to the blood, and adding slightly to glycogen stores in the liver and muscles. Such meals are typically high in carbohydrate, moderate in protein, and relatively low in fat because fat is more slowly digested than either carbohydrate or protein. When the time of exercise is known, mealtime can be predictable. For example, team meals are often scheduled three or four hours before competition.

However, an athlete may not have three or four waking hours before exercise, or may not know the time of exercise. Many athletes train early in the morning before going to work or school and do not awaken hours before they exercise. Rain delays or the length of previous matches may affect the start time of some sports, such as tennis, so these athletes would need to be cautious about eating too much too close to exercise. Because the amount of time before exercise and the amount of food or fluid consumed are related, guidelines have been developed for preexercise carbohydrate intake.

If the athlete is eating one hour before exercise, he should consume 1 gram of carbohydrate per kilogram of body weight (g/kg). Similarly, two hours before exercise the suggested carbohydrate intake is 2 g/kg, whereas 3 g/kg can usually be tolerated three hours before exercise. For example, carbohydrate intake for a 150-pound (68 kg) person would be about 68 grams one hour before, 136 grams two hours before, and 204 grams three hours before exercise. A sample preexercise meal for each of these time frames is shown on page 51.

To avoid gastrointestinal distress as the time before exercise gets closer, athletes may find it beneficial to move from solid carbohydrate foods to semisolid or liquid carbohydrate. A plate of spaghetti with tomato sauce may be the appropriate amount and type of carbohydrate three hours before exercise, but a banana or sport beverage may be the carbohydrate foods that are best tolerated less than an hour before exercise. In the 60 minutes before the start of exercise, many athletes slowly consume carbohydrate-containing beverages.

Because the risk of gastrointestinal problems is real, athletes sometimes wonder whether they should not consume any food or beverages before exercise. Exercise performance, particularly endurance exercise, is typically decreased if performed on an empty stomach. This may be a result of low blood sugar, which results in hunger, irritability, and a lack of concentration. Fasting before exercise is not recommended, but it is sometimes a strategy used by wrestlers and other athletes before weight

SAMPLE PREEXERCISE MEALS

An athlete who weighs 150 pounds (68 kg) and is eating one hour before exercise can tolerate a meal of 68 grams of carbohydrate:

1 large bagel

1 teaspoon low-fat cream cheese

8 ounces orange juice

An athlete eating two hours before exercise can tolerate 136 grams of carbohydrate:

1 cup low-fat granola with raisins

1 cup nonfat milk

1 large banana

8 ounces of a sport beverage

A meal consumed three hours before exercise can contain 204 grams of carbohydrate:

2 bagel sandwiches (each sandwich is one large bagel, 4 thin slices of turkey, and 1 tsp. each of mustard and light mayonnaise)

1 large apple

2 individual packages of Fig Newtons (4 cookies)

8 ounces (240 ml) of a sports beverage

certification. Fasting reduces muscle glycogen. Once weight is certified, these athletes consume as much carbohydrate as they can tolerate before competition to try to restore as much muscle glycogen as possible.

Athletes are urged to determine the most appropriate amount, timing, and type of carbohydrate through the use of trial and error during training. Training is a time to experiment with preexercise carbohydrate intake. Athletes should then take the information gathered during training and apply it to the precompetition situation. Many athletes will need to adjust their usual intake before training to account for the stress of competition. For example, a marathon runner may not be able to tolerate the same volume or types of food normally consumed before training runs simply because of prerace gastrointestinal distress. It is common for athletes to feel a bit nauseous before competing.

During Exercise

Carbohydrate intake during exercise is beneficial when athletes need additional fuel while they are training or competing. The need is based on exercise duration. Prolonged endurance sports such as distance running, cycling, swimming, and cross-country skiing deplete muscle glycogen. These athletes can run out of stored carbohydrate, so it is beneficial to eat or drink some carbohydrate while exercising (Coyle, 2004).

> *If you're riding for more than an hour at a time, you need some kind of nutrition to keep you going. The food should be high in carbohydrates and low in fat. Energy gels and bars are good choices, but not all cyclists can tolerate these during their ride.*
>
> **Catherine Kruppa**, MS, RD, frequent speaker about sport nutrition and director of nutrition for US Diving

Carbohydrate intake during breaks in stop-and-go sports, such as soccer, basketball, and hockey, may be beneficial. Compared to prolonged endurance athletes, athletes in these sports do not need as much carbohydrate during exercise because the competition does not last as long. However, consuming some carbohydrate helps to stabilize blood sugar and reduces the athlete's perception of fatigue.

The general guidelines for carbohydrate intake during exercise are shown in table 4.2. They range from less than 30 grams per hour to up to 90 grams per hour. For athletes other than prolonged endurance and ultraendurance athletes, the general recommendation for carbohydrate consumption during exercise is 30 to 60 grams per hour. As a point of reference, 8 ounces (240 ml) of a traditional sport beverage contains approximately 15 grams of carbohydrate.

After choosing the recommended range for the sport, each athlete should use trial and error to determine how much works best, keeping the following points in mind:

- Nausea, vomiting, abdominal cramping, gas, or diarrhea can occur if too much carbohydrate is consumed.
- Most sport beverages are formulated to be 6 to 8 percent carbohydrate because this concentration can be tolerated by most people.
- The maximum absorption of carbohydrate is approximately 1 gram per minute, or 60 grams per hour.
- Distance runners tend to have more gastrointestinal stress during exercise than distance cyclists.
- What works well during training will likely need to be adjusted for competition because training can never simulate the stress of competition.
- Carbohydrate may be consumed in the form of drinks, gels, or foods; some of the more popular carbohydrate sources used during exercise are bananas, soft cookies such as Fig Newtons, energy bars low in fiber and fat (less than 4 grams of each), sport gels, and sport beverages (6 to 8 percent carbohydrate).

It cannot be emphasized enough that the general guidelines must be fine-tuned by each athlete, and experimenting with various types and amounts of carbohydrate during training is critical. Some athletes love gels and others cannot tolerate them. One of the biggest mistakes that an athlete can make is to consume a food or beverage for the first time during competition.

TABLE 4.2   Optimizing Carbohydrate Intake During Exercise

Event	Energy cost	Recommended intake of carbohydrate for optimal performance	Carbohydrate type
Maximal exercise lasting less than 45 min (Cycling sprints; most swimming events; most running events—including 10-km run)	>18 kcal/min	None required	
Maximal exercise lasting about 45-60 min (Cycling, 1-km time trials; intense basketball game; soccer, one period)	14-18 kcal/min	Less than 30 g/h	Glucose, sucrose, maltose, maltodextrins, amylopectin, fructose, galactose, isomaltulose, trehalose, amylose
Team sports lasting ~90 min (Soccer match)	5-10 kcal/min	Up to 50 g/h	Glucose, sucrose, maltose, maltodextrins, amylopectin, fructose, galactose, isomaltulose, trehalose, amylose
Submaximal exercise lasting more than 2 h (Recreational tennis match; recreational cycling; hiking and orienteering)	5-7 kcal/min	Up to 60 g/h	Glucose, sucrose, maltose, maltodextrins, amylopectin, fructose, galactose, isomaltulose, trehalose, amylose
Near-maximal and maximal exercise lasting more than 2 h (Marathon run; cycling, individual pursuit; competitive tennis match; 50-km ski race)	7-10 kcal/min	50 to 70 g/h	Glucose, sucrose, maltose, maltodextrins, amylopectin
Ironman triathlon, Tour de France stage races	10-14 kcal/min	60 to 90 g/h	May be achieved only by intake of multiple types of carbohydrate: glucose, fructose, sucrose, maltodextrins, amylopectin

Reprinted, by permission, from A. Jeukendrup, 2007, *Carbohydrate supplementation during exercise: Does it help? How much is too much?* Gatorade Sports Science Institute, SSE # 106. Retrieved October 6, 2008 from, www.gssiweb.com/Article_Detail.aspx?articleid=757&level=2&topic=15.

After Exercise

The recovery period begins as soon as exercise ends. One goal is to restore the muscle glycogen that was used during exercise. Both the amount and timing of carbohydrate intake will influence how fast and how much muscle glycogen is synthesized.

After exercise, muscle cells are more permeable to glucose. Hormones and enzymes are released that favor the uptake of glucose and the formation of glycogen. Studies have shown that a two-hour delay in carbohydrate consumption can substantially reduce the rate at which glycogen is resynthesized (Ivy, Katz, Cutler,

Sherman, & Coyle, 1988). Therefore, carbohydrate intake should begin as soon as possible after exercise and no later than one hour after exercise. To ensure rapid recovery, athletes should consume 1 to 1.5 grams of carbohydrate per kilogram of body weight during the first 30 minutes. For example, a 154-pound (70 kg) athlete should consume approximately 70 to 105 grams of carbohydrate in the half hour immediately after exercise. Carbohydrate consumption should continue at least every two hours for the next four to six hours (American Dietetic Association, Dietitians of Canada, & the American College of Sports Medicine, 2009). The initial foods or beverages should be followed by substantial snacks and, within the six-hour period, a high-carbohydrate meal.

Some carbohydrate foods raise blood sugar quickly, which is an advantage immediately after exercise. Examples of such foods include many sport beverages, chocolate milk, granola bars, sugared cereals, white bread, bagels, and soft drinks. These foods make good after-exercise snacks. The effect that various carbohydrate foods have on blood glucose level is discussed in the sidebar Use of the Glycemic Index by Athletes below.

Full restoration of muscle glycogen stores takes approximately 20 hours. For athletes who train hard on a near-daily basis or are competing in events that are

USE OF THE GLYCEMIC INDEX BY ATHLETES

As athletes fine-tune their carbohydrate intake, they may look at a food's glycemic response. *Glycemic response* refers to the effect of a carbohydrate-containing food or beverage on blood glucose concentration and insulin secretion. Foods that have a high glycemic response elevate blood glucose rapidly, followed by a rapid rise in insulin. Both are beneficial for maximal muscle glycogen resynthesis immediately after exercise.

However, high-glycemic-response foods by themselves may lead to being on a sugar roller-coaster. In other words, blood sugar rises rapidly and the athlete feels a quick burst of energy. However, the sugar in the blood is moved quickly into the cells, and within a half hour or so the athlete may no longer feel energetic. More sugar is needed to feel energetic again. One way to get off the sugar roller-coaster is to eat a meal that has a mixture of carbohydrate, protein, and fat.

The glycemic index is a tool used by athletes (and diabetics) to estimate a carbohydrate food's glycemic response. In general, a high-glycemic-index food is made from highly refined grains, has added sugar, or is a starchy vegetable. Beans, legumes, dairy products, and some fruits have a low glycemic index. These foods are often eaten before a moderate to long exercise bout because they provide glucose to the blood slowly. Following are examples of the glycemic index of popular foods:

- **High glycemic index (greater than 85 out of 100):** Clif bar, GatorLode, corn flakes, Gatorade, Power Bar
- **Medium glycemic index (between 60 and 84):** Waffles, Met-Rx bar, bagels, white rice, pancakes, Powerade
- **Low glycemic index (less than 60):** Ripe banana, apple, beans and legumes

held over consecutive days, rapid and full restoration of muscle glycogen is vitally important. Those athletes competing in multiple events in a day, such as wrestlers and martial artists, need to restore muscle glycogen rapidly. This is especially true if they began the day with low glycogen stores as a result of fasting or other methods to make weight. These athletes need to eat or drink carbohydrate immediately after having their weight certified to try to resynthesize as much muscle glycogen as possible as fast as possible, but without upsetting their stomachs.

How Does an Athlete Carbohydrate Load?

Some athletes need to have the maximum amount of muscle glycogen possible. Carbohydrate loading (commonly referred to as carbo loading) is a procedure used to achieve this goal. It is appropriate for athletes in prolonged endurance events who exercise continuously for more than 90 minutes and for bodybuilders preparing for a contest. Athletes in other sports generally do not need to have maximum glycogen stores at the time of competition.

The basic principle behind carbohydrate loading is that exercise depletes glycogen and carbohydrate foods restore glycogen. Although this is widely understood today, it was new scientific information in the late 1960s (Bergstrom, Hermansen, & Saltin, 1967). The following procedure is known to maximize muscle glycogen stores and is used by many bodybuilders:

- Start the procedure seven days before the day of the competition.
- For the first three and a half days (starting seven days before the competition), exercise to exhaustion while consuming a very low-carbohydrate diet.
- The diet in the first three and a half days is nearly all protein and fat.
- Expect to feel light-headed and irritable and to have difficulty exercising during this time.
- In the three and a half days immediately before the competition, consume a high-carbohydrate diet, equivalent to at least 8 grams of carbohydrate per kilogram of body weight per day. Keep exercise to a minimum so glycogen will not be used.
- Because muscles have been starved of carbohydrate, once it is consumed, they begin to maximize glycogen stores.
- Nausea, bloating, stomach cramping, and gas are common and may be very uncomfortable.

The preceding procedure proved to be too difficult and risky for many athletes. In 1981 Sherman and colleagues tested a modified protocol. Instead of exercising to exhaustion, athletes tapered their exercise over the six days before competition (see table 4.3, page 56). Beginning on the seventh day before the event, dietary carbohydrate was reduced to 5 g/kg/d for three and a half days. This allowed some muscle glycogen to be restored for the next day's training, which reduced the risk of injury. In the three days before the event there was little exercise, but dietary

TABLE 4.3   Traditional Versus Modified Carbohydrate-Loading Protocols

TRADITIONAL CARBOHYDRATE-LOADING EXERCISE AND DIET PROTOCOL		
	Exercise	**Diet**
7 days before competition	Exhaustive exercise	Low carbohydrate[1]
6 days before competition	Exercise to continue depleting muscle glycogen	Low carbohydrate
5 days before competition	Exercise to continue depleting muscle glycogen	Low carbohydrate
4 days before competition	Exercise to the extent possible	Low carbohydrate
3 days before competition	Rest or very light exercise	High carbohydrate[2]
2 days before competition	Rest or very light exercise	High carbohydrate
1 day before competition	Rest or very light exercise	High carbohydrate
MODIFIED CARBOHYDRATE-LOADING EXERCISE AND DIET PROTOCOL		
	Exercise	**Diet**
6 days before competition	90 minutes training at 70% $\dot{V}O_2$max	Moderate carbohydrate[3]
5 days before competition	40 minutes training at 70% $\dot{V}O_2$max	Moderate carbohydrate
4 days before competition	40 minutes training at 70% $\dot{V}O_2$max	Moderate carbohydrate
3 days before competition	20 minutes light training	High carbohydrate[4]
2 days before competition	20 minutes light training	High carbohydrate
1 day before competition	Rest	High carbohydrate

Darker-gray area is depletion stage, and lighter-gray area is repletion stage.

[1]Low-carbohydrate diet is defined as 10% of total energy intake as carbohydrate. It consists of protein and fat foods and only a small amount of juice or other carbohydrate foods.

[2]High-carbohydrate diet is defined as 90% of total energy intake as carbohydrate. It consists of all carbohydrate foods, some of which naturally contain protein. Foods containing fat or foods prepared with fat are not allowed. This diet is very high in fiber.

[3]Moderate-carbohydrate diet is defined as 5 grams of carbohydrate per kilogram of body weight.

[4]High-carbohydrate diet is defined as 10 grams of carbohydrate per kilogram of body weight.

Reprinted, by permission, from M. Dunford, 2005, *Current trends in performance nutrition* (Champaign, IL: Human Kinetics), 23.

carbohydrate intake was increased to 10 g/kg/d. The result was high muscle glycogen stores but the extremes—exercising to exhaustion and severe gastrointestinal distress—were eliminated. Today, most endurance athletes follow the less extreme protocol because it better fits their training and the results are excellent.

The Short of It

- Carbohydrates are found in foods as sugars, starches, and fibers.
- The majority of carbohydrate consumed should be as whole grains, beans, vegetables, fruits, and nuts because these foods also provide many nutrients including fiber.

- At times, a sugary food or beverage is the best choice because the sugar is absorbed rapidly and provides a quick source of energy.
- An adequate carbohydrate intake daily is essential for athletes to replenish glycogen stores that have been reduced during rigorous training or competition.
- Many athletes do not consume sufficient carbohydrate daily, which leads to fatigue.
- Guidelines for the amount and timing of carbohydrate before, during, and after exercise have been established but must be fine-tuned by each athlete based on individual tolerances.
- Carbohydrate intake during prolonged exercise in the form of drinks, gels, or food helps to delay fatigue and maintain exercise intensity.
- Athletes need to consume some carbohydrate immediately after exercise as part of their recovery strategy.
- Carbohydrate loading is a procedure used by prolonged endurance athletes and bodybuilders to attain maximum glycogen stores before competition.

CHAPTER 5

Protein

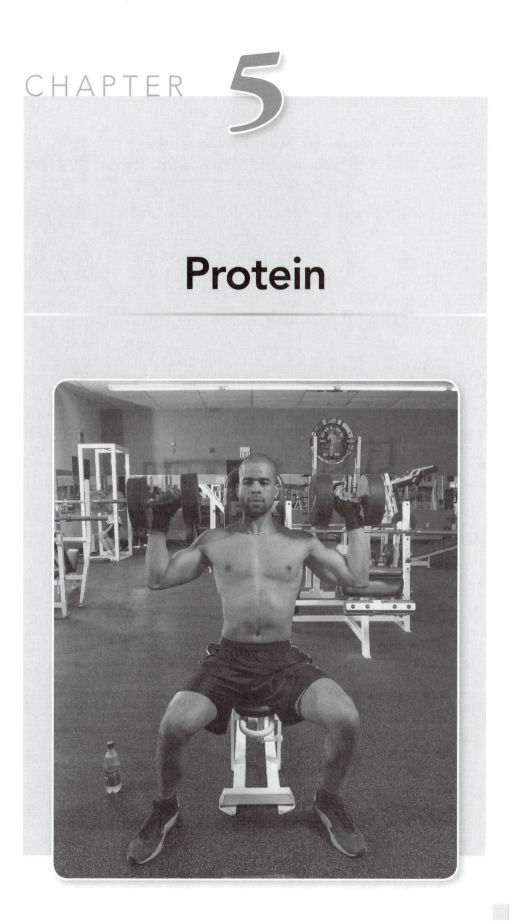

In this chapter, you will learn the following:

✓ Facts about protein and amino acids

✓ Foods that contain protein

✓ The amount of protein recommended for athletes daily

✓ Potential problems with taking in too much or too little protein

✓ Why some protein is needed after exercise

"Protein synthesis is a central problem for the whole of biology . . . ."

Francis Harry Compton Crick, British molecular biologist and codiscoverer of the structure of DNA in 1953

The first written record linking a high-protein diet to improved athletic performance is in Greece in the fifth century BC. Diets at the time were primarily vegetarian, and two athletes were reported to have increased their weight and strength by eating large quantities of animal flesh. Specific animal parts such as lion hearts and deer livers became popular not only for strength but in the hopes they would confer other attributes such as bravery and speed. The Greeks coined the word *protos* (meaning "first") and later *proteios* (meaning "of the first quality"), the forerunners to today's term *protein*. The search for the relationship between protein and improved athletic performance that began with the Greeks remains with us today.

What Are Amino Acids and Proteins?

Amino acids, which contain carbon, hydrogen, oxygen, and nitrogen, are the building blocks of proteins. There are 20 amino acids, nine of which must be obtained directly from protein-containing foods because they cannot be made by the body. These amino acids were once called essential amino acids, but the new term is *indispensable amino acids*. The remaining 11 amino acids are termed dispensable or nonessential amino acids because the body can manufacture them. In countries where food is plentiful, people likely consume the proper amount and types of amino acids and their bodies can build the proteins it needs.

amino acid—The basic unit of protein.

indispensable amino acids—Amino acids that must be obtained from food because the body cannot make them.

ligament—Fibrous tissue that connects bone to a joint or supports an organ.

tendon—Fibrous tissue that connects muscle to a bone.

The body makes many types of proteins. Although there are only 20 amino acids, the total number of amino acids in a protein is usually in the hundreds. The number and types of amino acids incorporated into the protein are responsible for its structure and function. For example, collagen is rigid because of the way the amino acids bind with each other. This makes collagen ideal for structural purposes such as cartilage, **ligaments**, **tendons**, bones, and teeth. In contrast, insulin is a protein-based hormone that must be small, stable, and flexible as it travels through the blood. Insulin contains only 51 amino acids, and the way the amino acids are bonded to each other makes it ideally suited for the job.

Importance of Protein

Food protein provides the amino acids necessary for making body proteins. For example, resistance training stimulates the genes in muscle cells to synthesize muscle protein. The muscle cells use amino acids to manufacture the muscle protein. Table 5.1 shows some of the many protein-based compounds made in the body.

TABLE 5.1   Functions of Proteins

Category	Function	Example
Hormones	Regulate body processes such as metabolism	Insulin, which regulates blood sugar level
Enzymes	Act as a catalyst for biochemical reactions	Lactase, which is necessary for the breakdown of milk sugar
Structural proteins	Give strength to muscle, skin, hair, and nails	Collagen, which is a strong fiber found in tendons and bones
Transport proteins	Assist the movement of compounds through the blood	Hemoglobin, an iron and protein compound that carries oxygen in red blood cells
Immune system proteins	Protect the body from the invasion of foreign particles	Antibodies, compounds formed in response to the presence of a foreign substance

Amino acids can also be used as an energy source. Under normal circumstances the body manufactures all the proteins it needs and then uses any extra amino acids provided in the diet as a source of energy. During temporarily stressful conditions, such as prolonged endurance exercise when glycogen stores are low, certain amino acids can be broken down to provide energy. The preferred energy sources for endurance exercise are carbohydrate and fat, but protein can be used as an additional energy source. Using protein as a source of energy under normal or temporarily stressful conditions is a normal metabolic response. However, of great concern is when caloric intake is too low over weeks and months and the body must use amino acids as a primary energy source. Under such conditions the body begins to break down **skeletal muscle** as a source of amino acids because it is not getting enough amino acids from food. If the starvation state continues, it also has a negative impact on the immune system.

> **skeletal muscle**—A type of muscle that powers movement; different from cardiac (heart) and smooth (blood vessels, organs) muscle.

Relationship of Protein and Energy

Anabolic refers to a metabolic process that builds complex molecules from simple ones. Such processes require energy. Athletes often refer to anabolism as tissue building, the tissue of interest being skeletal muscle. When amino acids are incorporated into skeletal muscle proteins, the process is anabolic. In contrast, when complex

Nutrition Bite

Is whey the way to go?

Whey and casein are specific types of proteins derived from milk. Whey is high in indispensable (essential) amino acids. Because of its amino acid composition, whey is absorbed quickly from the intestinal tract and is known as the fast-acting protein. In contrast, casein is slow acting because it is not absorbed as quickly as whey. Whey has been popular with strength and power athletes because there is some evidence that whey protein supplements increase muscle mass more than casein does.

As a protein source after exercise, either whey or casein supplements have been shown to increase muscle protein synthesis and aid in recovery. As a practical matter, athletes often ingest a protein supplement that contains both whey and casein so they ingest both fast- and slow-acting proteins. Similarly, milk or chocolate milk (for its added carbohydrate and taste) is a popular postexercise beverage that provides both whey and casein.

molecules are broken down into simple molecules, the process is termed catabolic. An example of catabolism is the breakdown of skeletal muscle to provide amino acids for use as energy.

Very simply stated, three things are needed in order to increase skeletal muscle:

1. Resistance exercise
2. Adequate calories
3. Adequate dietary protein

Resistance exercise provides the overload stimulus to which the muscles can adapt by increasing size and strength. Because muscle building is an anabolic energy-requiring process, daily caloric intake must be sufficient. Male athletes beginning a rigorous resistance training program typically need to increase caloric intake by up to 500 kcal daily; female athletes, to a lesser degree. It is estimated that a 1-pound (0.5 kg) increase in skeletal muscle requires the incorporation of about 100 grams of protein. This would be the equivalent of about 14 grams of dietary protein daily (assuming that a 1-pound increase in muscle mass would take seven days). This estimate assumes that the athlete is not using **anabolic steroids**, substances that are banned by nearly every sport governing body. Anabolic steroids may quickly and substantially increase skeletal muscle in some athletes, and their use likely requires a greater caloric and protein increase than that described in this chapter.

anabolic steroid—A hormone that promotes an increase in tissue size by increasing protein synthesis.

Sources of Dietary Protein

Protein is found in both plant and animal foods and dietary supplements. Animal-based protein sources include meat, poultry, fish, milk, milk products, and eggs.

Dried beans and **legumes**, nuts, seeds, grains, and vegetables are examples of plant-based proteins. Protein supplements, such as powders, beverages, and bars, are typically made from plant (e.g., soy) or animal (e.g., milk) proteins. Table 5.2 lists the protein content of various protein-containing foods.

legumes—A class of vegetables including dried beans, peas, and lentils.

TABLE 5.2   Protein Content of Selected Foods and Supplements

Product	Serving size	Protein (g/serving)
Light tuna packed in water	6 oz (170 g)	32.5
Protein bar	~2.5 oz (71 g)	28
Casein protein powder	1 scoop (32 g)	26
Whey protein concentrate	1 scoop (27 g)	24
Chicken (boneless, skinless breast)	~3 oz (85 g)	23
Whey protein isolate powder	1 scoop (25 g)	23
Soy protein powder	1 scoop (28 g)	23
Low-fat kefir	8 oz (240 ml)	14
"Weight gainer" powder	1 scoop (38 g)	14
Drinkable low-fat yogurt	8 oz (240 ml)	8
Egg white	2 large whites (66 g)	8
Soy nuts, dry roasted	1/4 c (1 oz, 30 g)	11
Low-fat (1%) chocolate milk	8 oz (240 ml)	8
Nonfat (skim) milk	8 oz (240 ml)	8
Peanut butter	2 tbsp	8
Almonds or walnuts	1/4 c (~35 g)	8

g = gram; oz = ounce; ml = milliliter; c = cup; tbsp = tablespoon

Nutrition Bite

What is the best source of protein?

Sasha Cohen, the 2006 Olympic silver medalist in ladies' figure skating, says, "I eat a variety of foods like vegetables, fruit, and beef for protein and iron." Jack LaLanne has long declared, "I only eat fish—no chicken, no turkey, just fish. I get all my protein from fish and egg whites." This raises the question: What is the best source of protein?

Like most areas of sport nutrition, there is room for individual choice in terms of what protein source is best. Athletes should consider the advantages and disadvantages of each. Beef contains protein, as well as iron and zinc, minerals that many female athletes lack in their diets. However, some cuts of beef are high in fat, and lean beef tends to be expensive. Similarly, fish and egg whites are excellent sources of protein, but some athletes would find such a diet too monotonous. Instead of focusing on the so-called best source, consider all the protein sources available.

What Is the Daily Protein Recommendation?

The recommended daily protein intake for sedentary or lightly active adults is 0.8 grams per kilogram of body weight (g/kg). For a 154-pound (70 kg) person this would be 56 grams daily. Recreational athletes who do minimal training may need as much as 1.0 g/kg, just slightly more than sedentary people. Based on data from research studies of trained athletes, it is generally recommended that endurance athletes consume 1.2 to 1.4 g/kg daily and that strength athletes consume 1.6 to 1.7 g/kg daily (American Dietetic Association, Dietitians of Canada, & the American College of Sports Medicine, 2009). Ultraendurance athletes may need up to 2.0 g/kg during periods of rigorous training and competition because of the body's use of protein as a source of fuel during prolonged exercise. As a rule of thumb, athletes likely need between 1.0 and 2.0 g/kg daily based on their training (see figure 5.1)

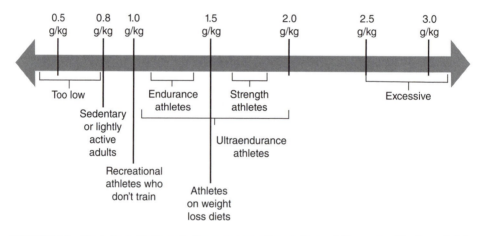

FIGURE 5.1 **Protein guidelines (g/kg = grams of protein per kilogram of body weight).**

These recommendations are a guideline; there is no way for an individual athlete to precisely know his or her protein need. Daily protein intake must be in balance with carbohydrate and fat intakes and within an appropriate caloric intake to meet the athlete's body composition goals. Consuming protein above 2.0 g/kg daily may be a practical problem because it does not allow for enough carbohydrate to restore muscle glycogen depleted by repeated days of heavy training. Consuming too great a carbohydrate intake may result in too low of a protein intake.

The need to properly balance protein intake with carbohydrate and fat intake has led to recommendations based on percentages of total caloric intake. In general, protein intake recommendations range from 10 to 30 percent of total calories, assuming that caloric intake is adequate to maintain body weight. Because of their need for a high carbohydrate intake, endurance athletes typically are advised to consume 10 to 15 percent of total calories as protein, whereas recommendations for strength athletes typically range from 15 to 20 percent. Some strength athletes prefer a higher-protein diet, equivalent to around 30 percent of total caloric intake, but that forces carbohydrate intake to be near the minimum amount recommended and restricts the fat content of the diet. A sample menu for a 150-pound (68 kg) person, which calls for 82 grams of protein (1.2 g/kg of body weight and 15 percent of total calories), is shown below.

An athlete's protein intake is closely tied to caloric intake. When caloric intake is low, protein intake tends to be low or marginally adequate. If caloric intake is adequate, most athletes consume protein within the general guidelines, or approximately 1.0 to 2.0 g/kg daily. Strength and power athletes may find that their intake exceeds the recommended 1.7 g/kg but is less than 2.0 g/kg daily. In other words, they may consume a bit more than recommended, but it is not substantially more because of the need for adequate carbohydrate. Surveys of bodybuilders report that protein consumption is 2.0 to 2.5 g/kg daily and, in some cases, up to 3.0 g/kg daily.

SAMPLE DAILY MENU CONTAINING APPROXIMATELY 82 GRAMS OF PROTEIN

Breakfast

1 cup orange juice

1 cup cooked oatmeal

1 teaspoon margarine

1 medium banana

1 cup nonfat milk

Lunch

2 slices wheat bread

4 oz (113 g) lean turkey

2 teaspoons mustard

15 baked potato chips

1 medium orange

1/4 cup trail mix (fruit and nuts)

Snack

12 ounces (360 ml) of a sport drink

2 large graham cracker squares

Dinner

1 1/2 cup spaghetti noodles

1 cup spaghetti sauce

1 cup cooked carrots

1 medium slice French bread

2 teaspoons margarine

Snack

8 ounces (240 ml) low-fat chocolate milk

Total protein from this menu is 82 grams, or 1.2 g/kg (grams of protein per kilogram of body weight), or 15 percent of total calories. This is based on a 150-pound (68 kg) athlete.

Is More Protein Better?

Over the years there has been much controversy over the amount of protein needed by athletes and whether high protein intakes are beneficial or detrimental. Bodybuilders often take in more protein than nutrition scientists recommend. They believe that the current recommendations may not be enough to support large, or maximum, increases in muscle mass or to repair the muscle proteins that are damaged by a large amount of resistance exercise. Some argue that a protein intake greater than 2.0 g/kg daily is beneficial because the precise amount of protein needed is not known. They suggest that it is reasonable to overshoot the mark to make sure there are enough amino acids to build the maximal amount of muscle tissue, recognizing that the excess will be used as energy. The practical problem with such an approach is that bodybuilders also want a low percentage of body fat, so they must control their caloric intake. If they consume large amounts of protein and sufficient carbohydrate to restore muscle glycogen, then their diets must be very low in fat to make sure that calories are not excessive.

The potential problem of greatest concern is that such high protein intakes result in excessive amounts of **nitrogenous waste**. The nitrogen portion of amino acids

⭐ SUCCESS STORY

Martin Gibala, McMaster University, Ontario, Canada

It seems as though Martin Gibala, PhD, has done it all. As a faculty member in the Department of Kinesiology at McMaster University in Ontario, Canada, Marty conducts laboratory research into the basic mechanisms that regulate energy provision in skeletal muscles. But Marty also conducts applied research that examines the impact of diet and

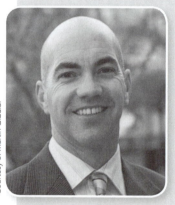

Courtesy of Martin Gibala.

training on athletic performance. That means he is equally skilled at understanding the details of amino acid metabolism in muscle cells and explaining what athletes should eat or drink to optimize their performance. No wonder he is a sought-after speaker at professional meetings and a frequent source of information for newspaper reporters.

McMaster University has emerged as a powerhouse of protein research, and Marty is quick to acknowledge the work of his internationally renowned colleagues Drs. Stuart Phillips and Mark Tarnopolsky, who often collaborate on his research studies. The group was one of the first to advocate the use of chocolate milk to promote muscle recovery after exercise. "We used to joke that we should conduct the 'tuna fish sandwich' experiment to show that eating real food was just as effective as supplements for stimulating protein synthesis after weightlifting (and a lot cheaper)," says Marty. "In the end Stu conducted studies with milk instead, and convincingly showed it was indeed very effective for stimulating muscle growth."

Consuming protein after weightlifting exercise is now a widely accepted practice. However, recent work by Marty and his colleagues suggests that protein is also important for endurance athletes and contributes to the recovery process by stimulating muscle protein synthesis (Howarth, Moreau, Phillips, & Gibala, 2009). This study highlights the ability of Marty's group to conduct elegant scientific investigations that address fundamental research questions but also have practical relevance for athletes. An editorial by noted protein researcher Dr. Nancy Rodriguez that accompanied the work concluded: "Howarth and colleagues have but scratched the surface of what promises to be an exciting area of investigative pursuits regarding the role of protein in a nutrient mixture for recovery from endurance exercise."

cannot be burned for energy so it becomes part of ammonia, which is toxic when accumulated. To avoid toxicity, ammonia must be converted to urea in the liver and be excreted via the urine. In the past, it was thought that high-protein diets

nitrogenous waste—Waste products, such as urine, that contain nitrogen.

would stress the liver and kidneys. Studies of athletes with normal liver and kidney function have not shown that high protein intakes are harmful (Phillips, Moore, & Tang, 2007; Poortmanns & Dellalieux, 2000). Those who consume high-protein diets are cautioned about the increased risk of dehydration, however. A high-protein diet requires more fluid to offset the increased urine excretion.

Which Athletes Get Too Little Protein?

Protein is too important of a nutrient to be overlooked; however, the majority of athletes consume a sufficient amount. The athletes who are at greatest risk for low protein intake are those who have eating disorders (see figure 5.2). Also at risk are those who have developed disordered eating patterns or who chronically undereat to keep their percentage of body fat and weight low. Some endurance athletes get so focused on a high-carbohydrate diet that they end up with a diet too low in protein. People with these issues need nutritional counseling because of potential health- and performance-related problems.

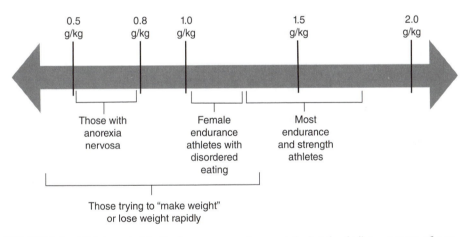

FIGURE 5.2 Athletes at risk for low or excessive protein intake (g/kg = grams of protein per kilogram of body weight).

How Does a Weight Loss Diet Affect the Need for Protein?

The amount of protein the body requires depends on caloric intake. When calories are restricted, the need for protein increases. The increase in protein may help to guard against the loss of protein from skeletal muscle, which would negatively affect performance and result in a decline in resting metabolic rate. As a rule of thumb, protein intake should be approximately 1.5 g/kg daily when restricting calories. Table 5.3 revises the sample menu shown earlier on page 65. The revised menu is higher in protein (119 g vs. 82 g) and lower in calories (2,023 kcal vs. 2,198 kcal). It also has less fat and carbohydrate than the original diet.

TABLE 5.3   Two Sample Diets Compared

Original menu	Revised menu (increased protein, decreased calories)	Comments
1 c orange juice	1/2 c orange juice	Portion size reduced by half
1 c cooked oatmeal	1 c cooked oatmeal	
1 tsp margarine	1 tsp margarine	
1 medium banana	1 medium banana	
1 c nonfat milk	1 c nonfat milk	
2 slices wheat bread	2 slices wheat bread	
4 oz (113 g) lean turkey	4 oz (113 g) lean turkey	
2 tsp mustard	2 tsp mustard	
15 baked potato chips	1/4 c soy nuts	Potato chips replaced with a higher-protein snack, soy nuts
1 medium orange	1 medium orange	
1/4 c trail mix (fruit and nuts)	1/4 c trail mix (fruit and nuts)	
	1 c nonfat frozen yogurt	Frozen yogurt adds protein
12 oz (360 ml) of a sport drink	12 oz (360 ml) of a sport drink	
2 large graham cracker squares	1 large graham cracker square	Portion size reduced in half
1 1/2 c spaghetti noodles	6 oz (170 g) cooked fish	Fish is a concentrated source of protein
1 c spaghetti sauce	1 medium baked potato	Potato goes well with fish
1 c cooked carrots	1 c cooked carrots	
1 medium slice French bread	1 medium slice French bread	
2 tsp margarine	2 tsp margarine	
8 oz (240 ml) low-fat chocolate milk	12 oz (360 ml) nonfat chocolate milk	Portion size is increased, which adds protein

Original diet: 2,198 kcal, 82 g protein (15%), 344 g carbohydrate (63%), 59 g fat (24%)

Revised diet: 2,023 kcal, 119 g protein (24%), 300 g carbohydrate (60%), 46 g fat (20%)

c = cup; tsp = teaspoon; g = gram; oz = ounce; ml = milliliter

Timing of Protein Intake

Studies suggest that the timing of protein intake is important. Exercise represents a catabolic condition because carbohydrate, fat, and in some cases protein are broken down to provide energy and muscle fibers are damaged. After exercise, a window of opportunity exists to help the body recover. It has long been known that consuming carbohydrate within the first hour after exercise helps to restore muscle glycogen.

In addition to carbohydrate, athletes should also consume protein in the first hour after exercise to help with muscle repair and growth.

The amount of protein needed after exercise is small, about 8 to 10 grams of an animal or soy protein. It is typically consumed with carbohydrate, which stimulates the release of insulin. Insulin is primarily involved with carbohydrate metabolism, but it also stimulates the uptake of amino acids into muscle cells. Popular drinks after exercise include low-fat chocolate milk, **kefir**, yogurt smoothies, and sweetened protein shakes, which provide protein, carbohydrate, and calories to support muscle repair, restoration, and growth.

kefir—A creamy yogurt-type drink.

Can Vegetarians and Vegans Get Enough Protein From Food?

Vegetarians do not consume animal flesh—meat, poultry, and fish—but may consume animal-based products such as eggs, milk, and cheese. Vegans do not consume any product derived from animals. It is usually recommended that vegan and vegetarian athletes who consume few animal products add 10 percent to protein recommendations to compensate for the lower absorption of plant proteins compared to animal proteins. For example, if the guideline suggests that an athlete needs 70 grams of protein daily, then a vegan athlete would be advised to consume 77 grams of protein daily.

> *Nothing will benefit human health and increase chances for survival of life on Earth as much as the evolution to a vegetarian diet.*
>
> **Albert Einstein**, physicist, known for his theory of relativity

Vegetarian athletes should include plant foods with a relatively high protein content, such as beans, particularly soybeans, and legumes. In the past it was thought that vegetarians needed to eat certain combinations of plant proteins at the same meal. Scientists currently believe that such strict timing is not necessary. However, vegetarians are encouraged to consume a variety of plant proteins throughout the day.

Are Protein Supplements Beneficial?

Protein supplements are heavily advertised particularly to strength and power athletes. These ads often emphasize that such athletes need more protein than the general population. Most ads do not mention that the majority of strength and power athletes meet their daily protein intake goals because their diets are relatively high in protein.

The bottom line is that protein supplements are no more or less effective than food proteins. In fact, most protein supplements are made from food proteins, such as egg whites, milk, and soy. Protein supplements are convenient, easy to transport, and can fit into an athlete's overall diet plan. The benefit to protein supplementation is likely the convenience, especially as resistance-trained athletes have become more focused on the timing of protein intake after exercise. The downside to excessive protein intake (as either supplements or food) is the possibility of low carbohydrate or excessive calorie intakes. As mentioned earlier, a high-protein diet also affects fluid balance and may increase the risk of dehydration.

One scoop (about 1 oz or 30 g) of most protein powders contains about 25 grams of protein, which provides about 10 grams of indispensable (essential) amino acids. These amounts match or exceed the amounts found in research studies to stimulate muscle protein synthesis (in the presence of resistance training and adequate caloric intake). In many cases, a scoop of protein powder contains about the same amount of protein and calories as 3 ounces (90 g) of roasted white meat chicken.

Most high-protein bars contain 25 grams each of protein and carbohydrate and some fat. Therefore, they contain more calories and more fiber than a liquid protein supplement. These may be beneficial to consume after workouts because athletes need some calories, carbohydrate, and protein after exercise. However, frequently snacking on high-protein bars may result in too high of a caloric intake over the course of a day. *Supplement* means "to add to," so athletes must consider how protein supplements fit into their overall diet plans.

> *For most healthy exercisers, including athletes, it is likely that proteins in normal meals will be sufficient to stimulate muscle growth, provided, of course, that the training stimulus is sufficient.*
>
> **Kevin Tipton**, PhD, University of Texas Medical Branch

The Short of It

- Adequate protein intake daily is essential for athletes.
- Athletes need more protein than sedentary people, but not as much as they might assume.
- In general, athletes need between 1.0 and 2.0 grams of protein per kilogram of body weight daily.
- For most athletes, protein recommendations can be met with food alone.
- Protein can be obtained from animal and plant foods and protein supplements.
- Protein supplements are convenient, and some athletes include them as part of their total protein intake.
- Protein intake must be balanced with carbohydrate and fat intake.
- A small amount of animal or soy protein after exercise helps in recovery.
- The need for protein increases when calories are restricted.

CHAPTER 6

Fat

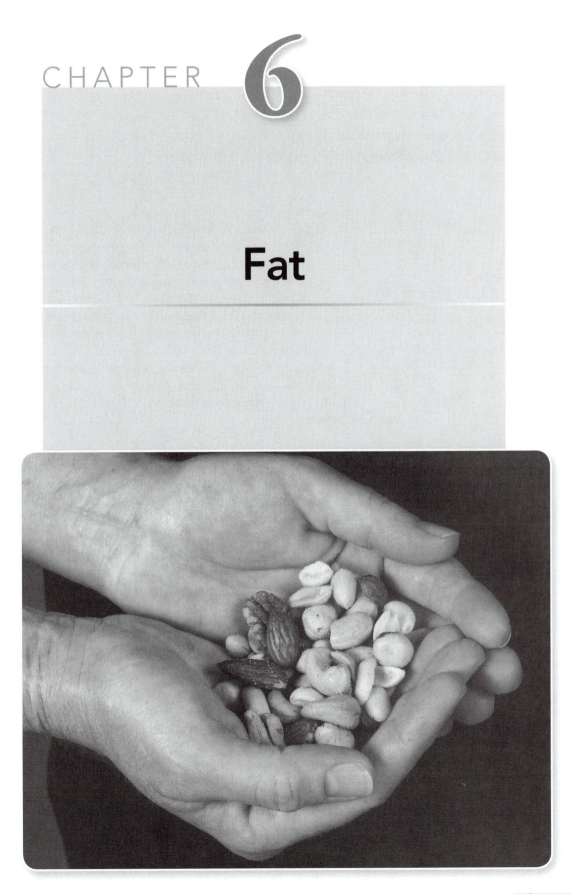

> "Cigarette sales would drop to zero overnight if the warning said, cigarettes contain fat."
>
> **Dave Barry**, American writer and humorist

"Consume a high-carbohydrate diet" is the take-home message of many magazine articles aimed at endurance athletes. But occasionally these same magazines run articles whose message is "Eat more fat." Why would highly respected magazines for trained distance athletes make a case for a higher-fat diet? Besides, isn't fat bad for athletes? To understand how much fat an athlete should consume, one needs to understand the nature of fat, the complexities of fat metabolism, and **macronutrient** balance.

What Is Fat?

Simply stated, a fat is a long chain of carbon molecules. The most frequently found fat in both the body and in food is the triglyceride. Of all the fat consumed in food, nearly 95 percent is triglycerides; the remainder is **sterols**, such as cholesterol and **phospholipids.**

macronutrient—A nutrient needed in a large amount, such as carbohydrate, protein, and fat.

sterol—A fat whose core structure contains four rings.

phospholipid—A fat that contains phosphorus and is predominantly found in cell membranes.

double bond—A chemical bond between two atoms that share two pairs of electrons.

A triglyceride is three fatty acids attached to a glycerol as shown in figure 6.1. All three fatty acids in the triglyceride may be the same. However, it is more common for the three fatty acids to be different.

Fatty acids are often classified based on their degree of saturation with hydrogen. A saturated fatty acid is completely saturated with hydrogen. A monounsaturated fat has one **double bond** so it is less saturated with hydrogen. Polyunsaturated fatty acids are those that have two or more double bonds between carbons so they are the least saturated with hydrogen.

Foods are typically categorized according to the predominant fatty acid found in them. For example, coconut oil contains about 92 percent saturated fatty acids. Other foods that are high in saturated fat include palm kernel oil (80 percent), dark chocolate (75 percent), butter (65 percent), and beef (45 percent). The sources of saturated fatty acids in the North American diet are typically foods containing either palm or coconut oils, such as snack foods and candy bars, or animal fat, such as whole milk, cheese, and other full-fat dairy products.

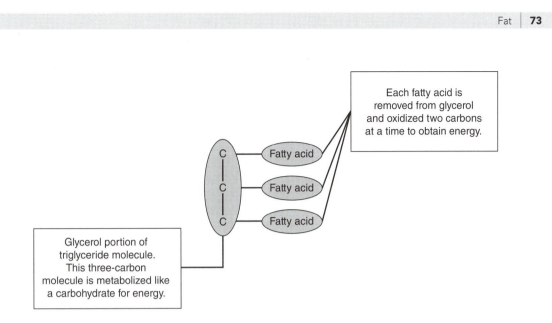

FIGURE 6.1   Triglyceride.

Reprinted, by permission, from D. Benardot, 2006, *Advanced sports nutrition* (Champaign, IL: Human Kinetics), 20.

Foods that contain primarily monounsaturated fatty acids are avocados (82 percent), olive oil (75 percent), canola oil (60 percent), almonds (65 percent), and peanut oil (50 percent). Oils such as corn and soybean are predominantly polyunsaturated fat (47 to 57 percent). Although fat-containing foods are categorized according to the primary fatty acid they contain, all foods contain a mix of fatty acids, as shown in figure 6.2.

The degree of saturation of the fatty acids consumed in food is an important health issue. Excessive intake of saturated fatty acids is a risk factor for heart disease. On the other hand, monounsaturated and polyunsaturated fatty acids have been found

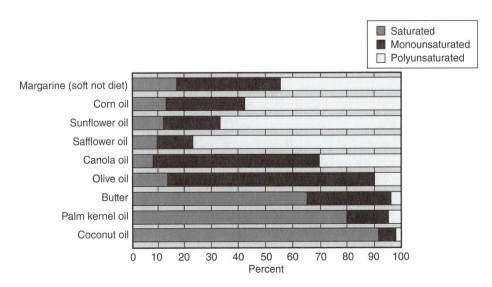
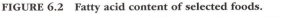

FIGURE 6.2   Fatty acid content of selected foods.

Reprinted, by permission, from M. Dunford, 2009, *Exercise nutrition, version 2.0* (Champaign, IL: Human Kinetics), 11.

Nutrition Bite

Sometimes it is easy to be fooled about the amount of fat or types of fat in a product. For example, most people consider granola a healthful food. Some granola bars and cereals have little sugar or fat added. Those brands are indeed healthful. However, many granolas have a lot of added fat and sugar. One popular brand of granola cereal contains 15 grams of fat in a half-cup serving, which is about the same amount of fat as in a small cheeseburger at a fast-food restaurant. Some of this fat is saturated fat. Granola bars can contain trans fat too.

It helps to read the food label to know for sure how much fat and the types of fat that are in the product. But to be realistic, it is important to also look closely at the serving size listed. For example, the label on a package of cookies may say 3 grams of fat, but that is the amount found in one cookie. If you know you would eat five cookies, then you are fooling yourself if you don't multiply that number by 5.

to decrease the risk of heart disease. It is a good idea to limit the consumption of saturated fatty acids. It is also wise to limit total fat intake to no more than 35 percent of total calories. In other words, people should not consume too much dietary fat and should make sure that most of that fat is not saturated.

How Is Fat Digested, Stored, and Utilized for Energy?

Fat digestion and absorption are complicated and time consuming especially when compared to carbohydrate. Complete digestion takes hours as the fat slowly moves from the stomach through the small intestine and into the blood. Athletes should not consume a large amount of fat too close to the time of exercise because it stays in the stomach and can cause discomfort when exercising, especially at moderate to high intensity. However, eating some fat can be helpful because the athlete's hunger is satisfied. For example, basketball players do not typically have much fat in their precompetition meals, but golfers may. Athletes need to balance the amount and timing of fat intake prior to exercise.

Triglycerides, which contain the fatty acids found in food, are attached to carriers and transported in the blood. Fat storage is typically high after a meal because hormones influence the triglycerides to be absorbed by fat cells, known as adipose cells. Fat can also be absorbed to a small degree by muscle cells.

When needed, the fat stored in adipose cells can be released and transported to other cells, including muscle cells. Once in the cells, fatty acids are moved to the **mitochondria**, the powerhouses of cells. The fat is then metabolized, and energy is produced.

mitochondria—Structures within cells that are responsible for the aerobic production of energy.

One of the benefits of endurance training is an increase in the number and size of mitochondria in muscle cells. This adaptation enhances the ability of some muscle fibers to use fatty acids as an energy source.

⭐ SUCCESS STORY

Rob Skinner, Director of Sports Nutrition, University of Virginia

Rob Skinner, MS, RD, CSSD, CSCS, is currently the director of sports nutrition at the University of Virginia. Previously, Rob was at the Georgia Institute of Technology. There he worked with a basketball player, a freshman athlete who was Muslim. Rob's story is a classic example of having everyone working toward the common goal of keeping an athlete healthy and playing. Here is Rob's account:

"An athletic trainer from another school and I were talking about Ramadan and how to help student-athletes compete during a time of fasting. I started wondering about the Muslim athletes at Georgia Tech. Ramadan fell right at the beginning of basketball season, and I was concerned about how performance during the month of fasting might be affected.

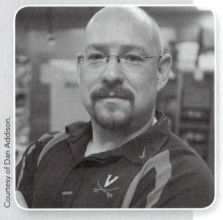

Courtesy of Dan Addison.

"My athlete shared his past experiences and how important it was to celebrate this holy month. We developed a feeding schedule to make sure he received adequate recovery nutrition after fasting during daylight hours. The athletic trainer made sure that fluids and food were available at practices so that once the sun went down, the athlete could stop practice and 'break fast,' giving him energy to participate in practice. The strength coach modified the workout and altered workout times as the month went on to give him the optimal time to recover from fasting during the day. As the nutritionist, I packed food from training table, so there was adequate nutrition available in his dorm room at night, including shakes, bars, and vitamin supplementation. Other than the athlete himself, the most important person was the head coach, Paul Hewitt. He treated this seriously, knew that nutrition played an integral role in the health and performance of his players, and fostered a team approach to the situation."

Coach Hewitt said, "Rob did a great job in educating the coaching staff, trainers, and strength coach on what needed to be done to keep my player on the court during our competitive season. The plan he put together was detailed but simple, and having a plan meant having success."

How Is Fat Used During Rest and Exercise?

At rest, approximately 75 to 80 percent of the energy needed to keep the body alive comes from fat. The remainder comes primarily from carbohydrate. Although the percentage is high, the total amount of energy being used is low. For example, during rest the amount of energy used by a 145-pound (66 kg) person is about 90 kcal per hour. Fat provides about 72 of the 90 kcal, or 80 percent. However, 72 kcal is a small amount, equivalent to less than 2 teaspoons of oil.

Fat is also the predominant fuel source during **low-intensity exercise**. Walking two miles in one hour is an example of low-intensity exercise. When compared to rest, the percentage of energy coming from fat during low-intensity exercise will decline from approximately 75 to 80 percent to approximately 60 percent. However, the amount of energy used will be twice the amount used at rest. Fat is the source of most of the energy both at rest and during low-intensity exercise. However, there is a big difference between the amount of fat (and therefore calories) used when resting and the amount used during low-intensity exercise.

low-intensity exercise—A low level of work during exercise, or less than 50 percent of maximal oxygen consumption ($\dot{V}O_2$max).

moderate-intensity exercise—A moderate level of work during exercise, or between 51 and 74 percent of maximal oxygen consumption ($\dot{V}O_2$max).

As exercise becomes **moderately intense**, such as brisk walking, the percentage of energy derived from fat declines to around 25 percent. It becomes more efficient for the body to use carbohydrate than fat as exercise intensity increases.

In the case of prolonged endurance activity, such as running a marathon at a steady pace, there is a slight change in fuel usage as muscle glycogen stores are depleted. Under this circumstance there is a slight increase in fat usage, a slight decrease in carbohydrate usage, and an increase in the use of certain amino acids for energy. This is the body's way of adapting to the decline in muscle glycogen stores during endurance exercise, which represents a temporary starvation state. The bottom line is that the body uses more or less fat based on the intensity and duration of exercise.

Nutrition Bite

"I'm in ketosis and burning lots of body fat. Isn't that a good thing?"

Low-calorie and low-carbohydrate but high-protein and high-fat diets (such as the Atkins diet) are popular for rapid weight loss. One of the expected side effects of such diets is ketosis. Normally, the brain relies on glucose for energy, but when a person consumes very little dietary carbohydrate, daily glucose is in short supply. The brain begins to rely on ketones, compounds produced when fat is broken down. An excessive rise in ketones is known as ketosis. Ketosis is not the same as ketoacidosis, a dangerous medical condition for those with uncontrolled diabetes.

During the first four weeks of ketosis, weight loss is rapid and it may seem as though the fat is melting away. Such a diet is not typically recommended for athletes because of the negative effect such a low carbohydrate intake would have on training. Muscle glycogen stores would be rapidly depleted and not restored. A low caloric intake would affect training volume and intensity. The disadvantages would likely outweigh the advantages.

Do Men and Women Metabolize Fat Differently?

In general, fat metabolism in men and women is similar because the biochemical processes are the same for all humans. However, there are some subtle differences due to hormones. Endurance-trained women use slightly more fat and slightly less carbohydrate than endurance-trained men do. It is important for both male and female endurance athletes to consume a diet that is high in carbohydrate but not too low in fat. A very low-fat diet may not adequately replenish the fat in muscle cells, an important source of fuel for endurance and ultraendurance athletes, especially women.

Is a High-Fat Diet Beneficial for Endurance Athletes?

As mentioned at the beginning of this chapter, some researchers are studying the effects of a high-fat diet in well-trained distance runners and cyclists. The use of a high-fat, low-carbohydrate diet does result in a greater usage of fat at rest and during low- to moderate-intensity activities. However, these exercise intensities are lower than the intensity at which an endurance athlete would train and compete. Therefore, a high-fat, or fat-loading, diet would not likely enhance endurance performance.

What Does *Fat Burning* Mean?

One of the most popular terms used today is *fat burning,* and it is used in reference to both exercise and food. Unfortunately, the term has added to the confusion surrounding fat in food and fat in the body.

Much has been written about exercising in the fat-burning zone. It is true that a person burns a higher percentage of fat during low-intensity exercise than during higher-intensity exercise. However, the total amount of fat used when exercising at low intensity is small. The most important factor in losing body fat is the total amount of calories used—not the intensity of the exercise or the amount of fat used during exercise.

Foods are typically described as fat burning based on their effect on resting metabolic rate (RMR). All foods temporarily raise RMR because it takes some energy to digest them. Protein has more of an effect on RMR than carbohydrate does, whereas the effect of fat is negligible. This had led some people to think that lean-protein foods, such as egg whites, poached fish, and baked chicken breasts, are fat burning. The truth is that the overall effect on the number of calories burned by digesting lean protein foods is small.

Many foods are advertised as fat burning—green tea, grapefruit, and hot peppers are a few examples. Nearly all foods advertised as fat burning contain a chemical compound that, when isolated in a laboratory, temporarily increases RMR. But there is not much of that chemical in these foods naturally, so eating any of them would have little effect on body weight.

No diet will remove all the fat from your body because the brain is entirely fat. Without a brain, you might look good, but all you could do is run for public office.

George Bernard Shaw, Irish writer (1856-1950)

What Is the Daily Recommendation for Fat?

Two factors determine the amount of fat in the athlete's diet—caloric intake and macronutrient balance. All three macronutrients—carbohydrate, protein, and fat—are important, but carbohydrate and protein needs are usually established first. This is not to say that carbohydrate and protein are more important than fat, but rather, that they take higher priority than fat because of their impact on performance. For example, sufficient carbohydrate is needed to restore glycogen and sufficient protein is needed to build or maintain muscle mass, both of which support training and recovery.

For the general population, the daily recommended intake of fat is 20 to 35 percent of total caloric intake. Many athletes also consume fat within this range. However, carbohydrate and protein recommendations for athletes are usually calculated on a gram-per-kilogram-of-body-weight (g/kg) basis rather than a percentage-of-total-calories basis, and combining the two methods can be confusing. To remain consistent with other macronutrient recommendations, a guideline for daily fat intake for athletes is approximately 1.0 g/kg daily. However, it may be lower (e.g., 0.65 g/kg) when fat intake is being restricted as part of a short-term weight loss plan, such as a bodybuilder's precontest preparation. It may also be higher (e.g., 2.0 to 3.0 g/kg) during rigorous training, such as an ultraendurance athlete's high-volume training period.

Table 6.1 compares daily fat intake for three elite athletes, each in a different sport and of a different body weight. In this example, the percentage of total calories coming from fat daily ranges from 20 to 23 percent, or approximately 1.0 g/kg. These athletes' diets tend to be lower in fat compared to the diets of sedentary people because their carbohydrate and protein needs are higher. This should not be interpreted to mean that athletes' diets *must* be low in fat; rather, that they often are.

essential fatty acids—Fatty acids that must be consumed in food because the body cannot make them.

Some athletes get too focused on consuming a very low-fat diet, which negatively affects their health and performance. Some fat is needed every day to provide the **essential fatty**

TABLE 6.1 Comparison of Fat Intake of Three Elite Runners

	Sprinter (100 m)		Middle-distance runner (1,000 m)		Long-distance runner (marathon)	
Height	190 cm	6'3"	180 cm	5'11"	165 cm	5'5"
Weight	88 kg	194 lb	68 kg	150 lb	56 kg	123 lb
Daily CHO intake	6 g/kg	528 g	7 g/kg	476 g	8 g/kg	448 g
Daily protein intake	1.7 g/kg	150 g	1.6 g/kg	109 g	1.4 g/kg	78 g
Daily fat intake	1 g/kg	88 g	1 g/kg	68 g	1.1 g/kg	61 g
Daily caloric intake	3,504 kcal		2,952 kcal		2,653 kcal	
% CHO intake	60		64		68	
% protein intake	17		15		12	
% fat intake	23		21		20	

m = meter, cm = centimeter, kg = kilogram, lb = pound, CHO = carbohydrate, g = gram, kcal = kilocalorie

acids and the fat-soluble vitamins A, D, E, and K. Too great a restriction of fat over time can result in **fat phobia**, a reduction in the manufacture of some hormones, and inadequate replenishment of fat in muscle cells. A very low-fat diet also does not satisfy hunger, which can lead to binge eating or overeating at the next meal or snack.

> **fat phobia**—A fear of consuming fat in food.

Some elite athletes have found it beneficial to increase the fat in their diets during periods of rigorous training. These athletes need a lot of calories every day, often more than 5,000 kcal. A high-carbohydrate diet at this calorie level means that these athletes also consume a lot of fiber, which leads to many bowel movements daily. By replacing some carbohydrate foods with foods that contain heart-healthy fat, such as oils, they lower the amount of fiber they ingest. When it comes to fat, athletes do not want a diet that is too low or too high.

> *The term "fat phobia" became popular in the early '90s when severely restricting fat intake was a common trend among athletes. I've noticed this trend resurfacing in many sports, and it's a serious problem for some people.*
>
> **Michelle Rockwell**, MS, RD, CSSD, sport nutrition consultant with rkteamnutrition.net

Sources of Fat

Fat and oil, such as butter, margarine, mayonnaise, and vegetable oils, are obvious sources of fat. When these types of fat are added to foods, they are often referred to as hidden fat because their presence may not be as obvious. Snack foods such as chips, crackers, candy, and cookies often contain fat. Reading the food label is one way to know the amount and source of fat in the product. Avocadoes, nuts, and seeds have a high proportion of fat, but they also contain carbohydrate and protein. Meat, fish, poultry, and dairy products, such as milk and cottage cheese, typically

TABLE 6.2   Strategies for Reducing Fat and Caloric Intake

Strategy	Foods	Fat (g)	Energy (kcal)	Fat savings (g)	Caloric savings (kcal)
Less fat in food preparation	Baked chicken vs. fried chicken (6 oz)	6 vs. 14	260 vs. 386	8	126
Adding less fat to food	1 tbsp vs. 3 tbsp margarine on a baked potato	11 vs. 33	101 vs. 303	22	202
Nonfat vs. full-fat foods	Fat-free sour cream vs. full-fat sour cream (2 tbsp)	0 vs. 5	24 vs. 51	5	27*
Smaller portion size	Starbucks Tall (12 oz, 360 ml) vs. Grande (16 oz, 489 ml) Double Chocolaty Chip Frappuccino Blended Crème Whip	14 vs. 19	380 vs. 510	5	130

*When the fat is removed, more carbohydrate is added typically in the form of starch.

g = gram, kcal = kilocalorie; oz = ounce, tbsp = tablespoon

contain fat. Within these broad groups are products with greater or lesser amounts of fat. For example, 8 ounces (240 ml) of whole milk contains approximately 8 grams of fat, whereas there is just a trace of fat in nonfat (skim) milk.

Athletes who want to reduce their fat and caloric intakes may want to focus on using less fat in food preparation, adding less fat to food, choosing low-fat or nonfat versions of foods, and reducing portion size. As shown in table 6.2, these four strategies can substantially reduce the amount of fat and calories in the diet.

Are Some Fats Associated With Health Risks?

In addition to knowing the amount of fat in food, it is wise to know the types of fat in foods. For health reasons, experts recommend that people limit the intake of saturated fatty acids, trans fatty acids, and cholesterol because they increase the risk of heart disease. Recall that saturated fat is fully saturated with hydrogen. It is found in animal products and palm and coconut oils. Trans fat is monounsaturated or polyunsaturated fat that has hydrogen added through a process called hydrogenation. Many snack foods contain trans fat because such fat helps products stay fresh longer. Cholesterol is a fatlike substance that is found only in animal foods.

Excessive intake of saturated fat and trans fat stimulates the liver to produce more low-density lipoproteins (LDL). LDL is a cholesterol carrier that tends to deposit excess cholesterol in arteries. Limiting dietary cholesterol intake to less than 300 milligrams daily is also recommended because in some people excess dietary cholesterol results in more blood cholesterol. Unfortunately, these kinds of fat have been labeled bad, an oversimplification of a very complicated issue.

Conversely, some types of fat are labeled as good, to indicate that they have been found to reduce the risk of heart disease. Examples are monounsaturated fat such as olive oil, polyunsaturated fat such as safflower and corn oils, and omega-3 fat found in nuts, flaxseed, green leafy vegetables, and cold-water fish.

From a practical perspective, many people need to reduce their total dietary fat intake daily because fat contributes to excessive caloric intake, which leads to overweight and obesity. In reducing their total fat intake, they typically also reduce their intake of saturated fat and trans fat and cholesterol, especially if they reduce the intake of animal fat and snack foods. The lower fat intake can also lead to weight loss.

However, people should not assume that heart disease risk is low if they are not overweight or obese. Athletes and others who are not overweight may have a high blood cholesterol level that could be lowered by changing the type of fat consumed. In all matters of health and disease risk, individual assessment is needed.

The Short of It

- Fat is an essential nutrient.
- Fat is the primary source of energy for the body at rest and during low- to moderate-intensity activity.

- Athletes need to balance fat intake with carbohydrate and protein intake.
- Too much dietary fat as well as too little can be detrimental to health.
- Athletes may need to limit fat, but they should not try to eliminate it from the diet.
- An excessive intake of some types of fat, such as saturated fat, increases the risk of heart disease.

CHAPTER **7**

Vitamins

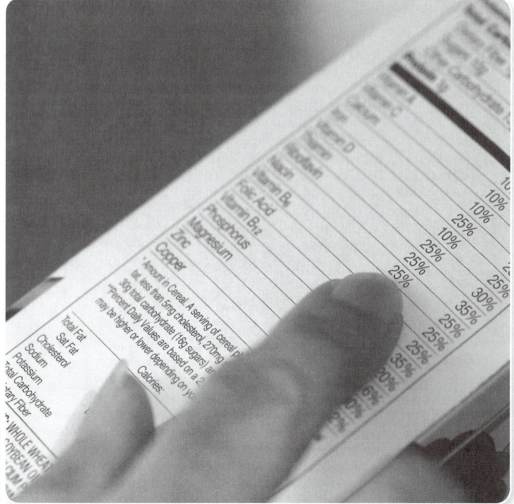

In this chapter, you will learn the following:

✓ Basic information about vitamins including how they function
✓ Recommendations for daily intake for 13 vitamins
✓ Food and supplement sources of vitamins
✓ The two major reasons athletes do not consume enough vitamins

"A nickel's worth of goulash beats a five dollar can of vitamins."

Martin H. Fischer, German-American physician and writer (1879-1962)

At the 2000 Sydney Olympic Games, all medal winners and some randomly selected athletes were required to provide urine samples and list any substances they had taken in the previous three days. After the Games were over, the data were analyzed and the authors concluded that there is "an unhealthy fixation amongst athletes in regards to vitamins. Athletes have now developed the same mind-set about vitamin supplements as they do about anabolic steroids, believing that their use is beyond question" ("Legal Drug Running," 2002).

The lead author of the study, Brian Corrigan, MD, said, "This is a big wake-up call. I think the results will shock a lot of people. The scary thing is this is what they took in three days. What they took in the months leading up to the Games is anyone's guess. They are mad, they are drug abusers. The amount of vitamin and minerals and supplements they take is crazy" ("Legal Drug Running," 2002).

One of the stars of the Games, 400-meter gold medal winner Cathy Freeman, spent $3,480 on vitamins and supplements from health food stores in the four months before the Games ("Legal Drug Running," 2002). Her spending was not considered unusual compared to that of her fellow competitors. The majority of the athletes assessed at the 2000 Olympics took vitamin supplements, usually in high doses, and sometimes by injection. Vitamin supplement use among the world's elite athletes continues today. Their hope is that vitamins will help, but the concern is that they will hurt, and the reality may be that these athletes have the most expensive urine in the world.

What Are Vitamins?

Vitamins are carbon-containing compounds that are essential for proper physiological functioning. They are referred to as **micronutrients** because each vitamin is needed in a small amount—milligrams or **micrograms** daily. Thirteen vitamins have been identified as essential in humans.

Vitamins are classified as fat soluble or water soluble. The fat-soluble vitamins—A, D, E, and K—are stored in **adipose tissue** and the liver. The advantage of fat solubility is that daily intake of these vitamins can vary. When intake is low, stores can be reduced; when intake is adequate or high, stores can be replenished. Excessively high intake over

micronutrient—A nutrient needed in a small amount by the body.

microgram—One millionth of a gram.

adipose tissue—Body fat.

a long period is dangerous because storage capacity is exceeded and liver function is affected. The greatest risk of toxicity is from an excessive intake of vitamin A and D supplements.

The remaining vitamins are water soluble and include vitamin C and the B vitamins—thiamin (B_1), riboflavin (B_2), niacin (B_3), pyridoxine (B_6), cobalamin (B_{12}), folate, biotin, and pantothenic acid. Water-soluble vitamins have no designated storage site; rather, tissues reach a saturation point beyond which the vitamin is excreted via the urine. In contrast to fat-soluble vitamins, when intake is low, tissue levels are reduced because there are no stores to compensate for low intake. Thus, adequate amounts of water-soluble vitamins should be consumed daily. Excessive amounts of some water-soluble vitamins consumed as supplements can result in toxicities, but such cases are rare because the body's tissue saturation/urinary excretion system works well.

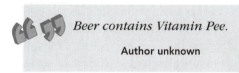

Beer contains Vitamin Pee.

Author unknown

The take-home message is that the problems are at the extremes. When intake is consistently too low over time, deficiencies of water-soluble vitamins can occur. Similarly, when excessive amounts of vitamins are taken over time, toxicities can occur. It has been documented in both athletes and nonathletes that low vitamin intake is typically a result of low caloric intake or a lack of vitamin-rich foods. It is highly unlikely that ingesting vitamins that naturally occur in food will result in toxicities; rather, excesses result from the intake of high-dose vitamin supplements, especially those that are readily absorbed. Such supplements have high **bioavailability**. These supplements are widely available for purchase and are frequently advertised to athletes and others who might be influenced by a "more is better" approach. *Caveat emptor*—Buyer beware!

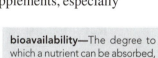

bioavailability—The degree to which a nutrient can be absorbed, metabolized, and used by the body.

How Do Vitamins Function?

Each vitamin has a unique biochemical role that cannot be fulfilled by another vitamin. Also, because each vitamin plays multiple roles, the effects of a single vitamin deficiency can be far-reaching. It is convenient to group vitamins according to their major functions, especially those that may affect performance. Therefore, vitamins are often categorized based on their roles in energy metabolism, as antioxidants, or in red blood cell production. The majority of studies of vitamins and exercise have been conducted in endurance athletes; nonendurance athletes are studied much less frequently.

Vitamins and Energy

The B-complex vitamins, particularly thiamin, riboflavin, and niacin, are involved in energy reactions. B vitamins are cofactors needed by the enzymes that regulate energy metabolism. Without vitamins, enzymes could not function and the body could not produce energy. However, the role of vitamins in energy production is indirect, not direct. In other words, vitamins do not directly produce the energy; they help the body release the energy that is contained in carbohydrate, fat, protein, and alcohol. A severe deficiency of the B-complex vitamins results in fatigue.

A severe deficiency of the B-complex vitamins in an athlete is unlikely. However, athletes do raise two interesting questions: Can a mild B vitamin deficiency affect energy production? Can increasing the amount of B vitamins increase energy production in well-nourished athletes?

Studies suggest that a short-term (less than three months), mild vitamin deficiency does not result in decreased performance, but long-term, moderate B vitamin deficiencies could (Lukaski, 2004). Such deficiencies are accompanied by low caloric intake and low intake of other nutrients. Thus, taking a B vitamin supplement can resolve the B vitamin deficiencies but not the low intake of carbohydrate or protein. When athletes are lacking B vitamins, they are usually more likely to benefit from treating the underlying problems, such as low calorie and carbohydrate intakes and consumption of vitamin-poor foods. By increasing the intake of fruits, vegetables, whole grains, beans, and lean protein foods such as fish and nonfat milk, athletes resolve all the nutrient-related problems, not just the B vitamin–related ones.

Consuming an excess of B vitamins does not result in an increase in the speed at which enzymes release energy or the production of more energy. Additionally, past the point of tissue saturation, the body will excrete excess B vitamins. An athlete who consumes a sufficient amount of the various B vitamins in food would not likely benefit from supplementation.

Vitamins and Antioxidants

When exercise lasts longer than seconds or minutes, energy is produced from carbohydrate, fat, or protein under aerobic ("with oxygen") conditions. The majority of the oxygen used in these reactions will eventually become water (H_2O), but approximately 4 percent will not. A small number of the oxygen molecules become free radicals, which are known as oxidants. Oxidants can damage cell membranes and tissues if they are not neutralized by antioxidants. An antioxidant is any compound that can slow or prevent the action of an oxidant. Some of the most potent antioxidants are vitamins, especially vitamin E. Oxidative stress occurs when oxidants outnumber antioxidants. The goal is to have antioxidants equal or slightly exceed oxidants (Urso & Clarkson, 2003).

Endurance athletes are at greater risk than others for oxidative stress because more free radicals are produced as the intensity and duration of exercise increases. Endurance training enhances the body's antioxidant defenses, but athletes must have enough antioxidants to counter the increased production of free radicals. This concern has naturally led to the study of antioxidant vitamin supplements, such as those containing vitamins A, C, and E, in endurance athletes.

There are few data that suggest that vitamin C supplements are effective for reducing oxidative stress in endurance athletes, and no data for the effectiveness of vitamin A supplements. Vitamin E is the most potent of the antioxidant vitamins, has the most potential to prevent damage from oxidants, and is the most studied. Unfortunately, the results of studies of vitamin E have been inconclusive, and experts do not agree about whether endurance athletes should consume vitamin E supplements. To date, about half of the studies report that oxidative stress is decreased with vitamin E supplementation, and half report no effect.

> **pro-oxidant**—A compound that induces oxidative stress.

A handful of studies report that vitamin E supplements increase oxidative stress because at high concentrations antioxidants act as **pro-oxidants** (Williams, Stobel, Lexis, & Coombes, 2006).

Nutrition Bite

In the mid-1990s taking vitamin supplements became popular to help lower the risk of diseases such as heart disease and cancer. First came vitamin E supplements to help prevent prostate cancer, then vitamin C to prevent various cancers, and supplemental B-complex vitamins and vitamin E to reduce the risk of heart disease. Vitamin supplement sales skyrocketed, and people began to believe that good health was just a vitamin pill away.

In the mid-2000s evidence began to emerge that lowering disease risk was not as easy as taking a vitamin pill. By mid-decade it had become clear that not only were these vitamin supplements ineffective for disease prevention, but some were actually harmful. In fact, some vitamin supplement studies were stopped to prevent harm to the participants.

Where do we stand now? At the end of the 2000s, most physicians are no longer recommending vitamin supplements as a way to prevent disease. However, they are sticking by age-old advice—eat right and exercise!

Until more definitive data suggest otherwise, experts recommend that athletes consume foods that are rich in antioxidant vitamins. This means eating a variety of fruits, vegetables, whole grains, nuts, and vegetable oils daily. Endurance athletes should assess their consumption of vitamin E–containing foods because surveys suggest that intake is often low. A common reason is the tendency of endurance athletes to consume a low-fat diet, which restricts their intake of vitamin E–rich foods. Excellent sources of vitamin E are vegetable oils, wheat germ, almonds, and sunflower seeds.

Vitamins and Red Blood Cells

Several vitamins are involved in red blood cell production, but the focus is generally on the two that play major roles— vitamin B_{12} and folate. Severe deficiencies of either vitamin can lead to anemia. In the case of vitamin B_{12} the most likely cause is low intake along with poor absorption, a condition most commonly seen in those over age 50. Another cause is the elimination of all animal products, the only naturally occurring sources of vitamin B_{12}. Such cases are rare because most vegans consume yeast or other products that are fortified with vitamin B_{12}. Deficiencies of folate leading to anemia are well documented, but the prevalence is lower now than before 1998 when mandatory folate fortification of cereals and grain products began in the United States.

Despite the low prevalence of vitamin B_{12} deficiency in athletes, some choose to inject vitamin B_{12} as an energy booster. There is no scientific evidence that vitamin B_{12} injections boost energy, delay fatigue, or increase red blood cell production in athletes who are not vitamin B_{12} deficient. In fact, the risks of such injections are likely higher than the benefits. Risks include soreness, swelling, development of **abscesses**, and contamination with banned substances.

abscess—A cavity filled with pus usually caused by a bacterial infection.

> *Although I do not know how this substance came into my body, it is possible that a shot of vitamin B_{12} I took sometime in April might have been the cause.*
>
> **Rafael Palmeiro**, professional baseball player, on the source of a banned steroid that was detected in his urine in the summer of 2005

How Much of Each Vitamin Is Recommended Daily?

For more than 60 years, scientists have been studying how much of each vitamin should be consumed daily. Vitamin recommendations are based on age, gender, and pregnancy. Table 7.1 lists the Dietary Reference Intakes (DRIs) for the 13 essential vitamins for male and nonpregnant females between the ages of 19 and 50. The DRIs were developed for healthy people who are moderately active, but they are also used as a guideline for athletes. In general, exercise does result in an increased need for vitamins, but the increased need would be small and would likely be met by the current recommendations. The DRIs include a margin of safety, and it is reasonable to assume that any vitamin losses caused by exercise would not exceed the safety margin.

Table 7.1 also lists the tolerable upper intake level (UL), an estimate of the highest level that can be consumed daily that is not likely to cause a health problem. Intakes above the UL can be toxic and are not recommended. It is legal to market and sell vitamin supplements containing amounts higher than the UL. *Caveat emptor*—Buyer beware!

Table 7.1 highlights several general issues about vitamins. Males need slightly greater amounts of vitamins A, C, B_1, and B_2 than females do. Vitamins A, D, K, B_{12}, folate, and biotin are needed in very small amounts, measured in micrograms. Smokers need more vitamin C than nonsmokers.

Upper levels have been established for seven vitamins. When the tolerable upper level is compared to the DRI, the magnitude of the difference can vary. For example, the UL for vitamin E is 67 times higher than the DRI, one of the reasons that vitamin E toxicity rarely occurs even though it is a fat-soluble vitamin. However, the differ-

TABLE 7.1   **Dietary Reference Intakes for 13 Essential Vitamins**

Vitamin	DRI—adult* male	DRI—adult* nonpregnant female	Tolerable upper intake level (UL)
Vitamin A	900 μg	700 μg	3,000 μg
Vitamin D	5 μg	5 μg	50 μg
Vitamin E	15 mg	15 mg	1,000 mg
Vitamin K	120 μg	90 μg	Not established
Vitamin C	90 mg (nonsmoker) 125 mg (smoker)	75 mg (nonsmoker) 110 mg (smoker)	2,000 mg
Thiamin (B$_1$)	1.2 mg	1.1 mg	Not established
Riboflavin (B$_2$)	1.3 mg	1.1 mg	Not established
Niacin (B$_3$)	16 mg	14 mg	35 mg
Pyridoxine (B$_6$)	1.3 mg	1.3 mg	100 mg
Cobalamin (B$_{12}$)	2.4 μg	2.4 μg	Not established
Folate	400 μg	400 μg	1,000 μg
Pantothenic acid	5 mg	5 mg	Not established
Biotin	30 μg	30 μg	Not established

*ages 19 to 50

DRI = Dietary Reference Intake; μg = microgram; mg = milligram

Data from: Institute of Medicine, 1998, 2000.

ence between the UL and DRI is much smaller for niacin (around 2.5 times higher), vitamin A (3 or 4 times higher), and vitamin D (10 times higher). Some athletes have experienced flushing and itching, known as a niacin rush, after taking a high-dose niacin supplement. This is an example of a health problem, albeit a temporary one, that can occur when exceeding the tolerable upper intake level.

Researchers agree that most athletes can obtain all the vitamins they need from food, but surveys show that many athletes do not because of poor food choices and low food intake. A low caloric intake resulting in a low intake of vitamins is a particular problem among female athletes who train rigorously but want to attain or maintain a low percentage of body fat. Distance runners and gymnasts are examples of athletes who are at risk for low calorie and vitamin intakes.

How Do Athletes Know Whether They Have a Vitamin Deficiency?

Vitamin deficiencies develop over time and progress from mild to moderate to severe. Assessing the athlete's usual dietary intake is a tool used to evaluate whether the athlete may have a mild vitamin deficiency. For example, it is safe to assume that vitamin intake is adequate if the athlete meets the DRI for each vitamin. If intake is less than recommended, it is harder to predict vitamin status. In some cases low intake can be offset by increased absorption or reduced excretion so a deficiency would not develop. In other cases, low intake could result in a mild deficiency because the body can only subtly change its absorption and excretion capabilities. To cover all possibilities, athletes should eat a sufficient amount of vitamin-rich foods daily. These foods are also likely to provide other nutrients that may be low in the diet, such as carbohydrate.

If vitamin intake is low over time, moderate deficiencies can occur as a result of low amounts in the tissues. Such deficiencies are difficult to detect, and athletes are unlikely to know that they have a moderate deficiency. It has also been difficult for researchers to determine the impact of moderate vitamin deficiencies on health and performance. The possibility of a moderate vitamin deficiency or a decline in performance are reasons athletes take daily multivitamin supplements. Such supplements provide the missing vitamins, but they do not address other nutrient deficiencies such as low carbohydrate or protein intake.

In times past, severe vitamin deficiencies were widespread, but in developed countries today diseases associated with vitamin deficiencies are rarely seen. A severe deficiency is unlikely unless food intake is severely restricted over time, such as in the case of an eating disorder. A vitamin deficiency could also result from a lack of exposure to sunlight caused by a constant use of sunscreen, being completely covered with clothing, or never going outside. People in these situations should consume foods fortified with vitamin D, such as milk. Severe vitamin deficiencies are also seen in alcoholics who get most of their calories from alcohol rather than food. Vitamins are needed to detoxify the alcohol, but the alcohol does not provide these nutrients. Once detected, severe vitamin deficiencies are easily reversed with the use of vitamin supplements.

Can Athletes Get Enough Vitamins From Food Alone?

Athletes can meet the daily recommendations for all the essential vitamins from food alone if they take in enough calories and eat a variety of vitamin-rich foods. Numerous surveys of athletes have shown that low caloric intake leads to low vitamin intake. This has been documented frequently in female distance runners, gymnasts, and ballet dancers and male wrestlers and jockeys. If athletes restrict their caloric intake, then the foods they eat must be **nutrient dense** or they run the risk of low vitamin intake. It is possible to consume low-calorie foods rich in vitamins. For example, a half-cup portion of cooked broccoli contains only 27 calories but 50 milligrams of vitamin C, which is 67 percent of the amount needed daily by nonsmoking females. Athletes who include fruits, vegetables, nonfat dairy products, lean protein foods, and whole-grain carbohydrates in their diets have a better chance of consuming enough vitamins without exceeding their desired caloric intake for the day.

nutrient dense—Containing a relatively high amount of nutrients compared to caloric content.

It is possible to consume a sufficient or excess amount of calories and still not meet daily vitamin requirements. Ironically, people can be overweight but malnour-

SUCCESS STORY

Mel Williams, Professor Emeritus, Ergogenics Expert, and Author

Mel Williams, PhD, is the preeminent figure when it comes to nutrition and performance. He is an international expert on ergogenic aids used by athletes to enhance performance and has written extensively about dietary supplements. He has long been concerned about athletes reaching for a magic pill or potion and believing that it can make up for a lack of training.

As a professor at Old Dominion University in Norfolk, Virginia, Mel researched the effects of many ergogenic aids, such as caffeine, creatine, and antioxidant vitamins. As new supplements became popular with athletes, sport nutritionists looked to Mel for answers to their questions—How does it work? Is it safe? Is it effective? Is it ethical? His extensive knowledge about nutrition as a way to improve athletic performance led to authoring a textbook, *Nutrition for Health, Fitness & Sport,* now in its ninth edition. Few in the field of sport nutrition today have not read his texts.

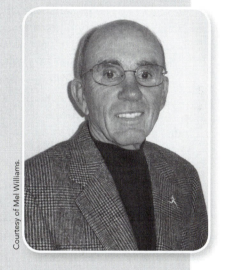

Courtesy of Mel Williams.

Christine Rosenbloom, PhD, RD, CSSD, nutrition professor at Georgia State University, says, "Early in my teaching career I was asked to develop a course on nutrition and physical activity. The first thing I did was choose my textbook—Mel Williams' *Nutrition for Health, Fitness & Sport*. The reasons I chose Mel's textbook were many, but the main reason was that he knew how to reach students—he just "got" them. Most texts cover the basics and have a separate chapter on ergogenic aids, but Mel knew that students didn't want to learn about protein in exercise without also discussing protein powders, amino acids, and creatine, so each chapter concluded with ergogenic aids. That kept students interested in the course and allowed for lively class discussions."

Mel Williams continues to inspire his peers both professionally and personally. In addition to a career that most academicians can only dream about, he has completed more than 100 marathons. He is the ultimate prof-runner, and many refer to him affectionately as the father of sport nutrition.

ished as a result of poor food choices. Athletes may consume enough calories but not enough nutrients, particularly if they rely on sweetened foods and beverages with low vitamin contents. Athletes can get all the vitamins they need from food, but they need to choose nutritious foods such as fruits, vegetables, beans, nuts, and whole-grain breads and cereals.

Sources of Vitamins

Vitamins are found naturally in foods, are added to foods when they are processed, and occur in supplements. Once the vitamin is absorbed, the body does not know whether it originally came from food or supplements. It is only looking for the chemical compound that it needs.

Dietary Sources

Vitamins are found naturally in a variety of foods. The advantages to obtaining vitamins from foods in which they naturally occur include a low likelihood of excessive intake, excellent absorption, and the consumption of other needed nutrients such as carbohydrate and protein (see table 7.2). Foods that are less processed tend to retain a majority of their vitamins; thus, a good piece of advice is to eat whole foods, or foods that are as close to farm grown as possible. Brown rice is unmilled or partially milled and is an example of a whole food, whereas white rice is extensively milled, which removes many of the vitamins.

White rice is also an example of a food that has vitamins added near the end of the manufacturing process. All grains and products made from them, such as breads and cereals, are required by law to add vitamins B_1, B_2, B_3, and folate in an effort to restore some of the nutrients lost. In this respect the processed and whole food have about the same amounts of those vitamins. However, not all lost vitamins, such as vitamin B_6, are restored, and other lost nutrients, such as magnesium, zinc, and fiber, remain lost.

Vitamins are also being added to foods even when the vitamin was not originally present. For example, milk is fortified with vitamin D. Sugared beverages are being

TABLE 7.2 Source of Vitamins Compared

Source of vitamins	Advantages	Disadvantages
Naturally occurring in food	• "Packaged" with other nutrients • Excellent absorption • Excessive intake unlikely	• Requires diet planning • Requires time and effort • Typically requires some cooking skills
Added to food (enriched or fortified)	• Adds vitamins to the diet • Some foods are more nutritious than the original • Intakes of vitamins that have been historically low are increased	• Not all vitamins removed during processing are restored • Other nutrients are lost and not restored • Competition for absorption
Supplements	• Adds vitamins that would otherwise not be consumed • Prevents or treats moderate to severe vitamin deficiencies	• Relatively easy to consume high or excessive amounts • Some are highly absorbable • Focus may be a single vitamin rather than total dietary intake • Unlikely to benefit well-nourished people and may increase risk for some diseases

pumped up with added vitamins, often vitamin C and B-complex vitamins. Breakfast cereal has long been a source of many added vitamins, and sport and energy bars have followed suit. The advantage to eating these foods is that they provide vitamins and are convenient, tasty, and popular. The disadvantages to eating these foods are that the vitamins may compete with each other for absorption and that these foods do not provide the range of nutrients that a variety of whole foods does.

Supplements

Vitamin supplements are an excellent way to treat and prevent severe vitamin deficiencies, although such deficiencies are relatively rare in athletes. A one-a-day type of vitamin has long been used as an insurance policy, providing an adequate amount of vitamins if the foods eaten do not. Many foods today are fortified with many vitamins, including cereals, energy bars, and meal replacement beverages. These foods represent similar insurance to one-a-day vitamin supplements. In the past, such practices were viewed as desirable or relatively harmless because of the role that adequate vitamin intake plays in preventing or delaying the onset of chronic diseases. Recently, concern has been expressed about the routine intake of vitamin supplements and highly fortified foods because of the increased risk for health problems. For example, some studies have shown that some hip fractures are associated with a high intake of retinol, which is preformed vitamin A found in some supplements. Some vitamins advertised to athletes contain high doses in highly absorbable forms, which increase the risk for excess absorption and toxicity. *Caveat emptor*—Buyer beware!

Nutrition Bite

Vitamin supplements are often advertised to athletes based on science. Here are some actual statements used to sell vitamin supplements. Consider whether they favor sales or science.

- *". . . is specifically designed for athletes of all levels including novice and professional."* This statement favors sales. Appealing to athletes of all levels calls into question how specifically the supplement is formulated. The vitamin needs of recreational athletes are unlikely to be higher than those of the general population, but endurance and ultraendurance athletes may need more antioxidants.

- *"Known to reduce the risk of neural tube birth defects, folic acid is needed for normal growth and development, and for red blood cell formation."* This statement favors science. These are well-documented functions of folic acid (folate).

- *". . . through this [vitamin] formulation we are able to enhance proper pH and particle sizes in our liquid multi, which maximizes absorption, which in turn maximizes effectiveness, which means optimum health. By rebalancing the body chemistry, toxins and other wastes are eliminated easily and safely via the kidneys."* This statement favors sales. Maximizing absorption does not mean that effectiveness is maximized, and vitamins alone would not have much of an impact on the body chemistry of a healthy person.

To properly determine the need for a vitamin supplement, by itself or as part of a multivitamin, an athlete must compare usual food intake to the DRIs for vitamins. *Supplement* means "to add to," so having baseline information about routine vitamin intake from food is important. Depending on the outcome of a dietary assessment, vitamin supplementation may be a consideration to prevent a long-term vitamin deficiency. Too often athletes skip the first step—assessment—and move immediately to the next step, which is deciding which supplement to buy.

> *The overwhelming focus on supplements isn't going to go away, but I would like to think that we could inspire athletes to be more interested in the benefits of wholesome foods.*
>
> **Louise Burke**, PhD, APD, FACSM, head of the department of sports nutrition at the Australian Institute of Sport

Those who use supplements when they are already obtaining enough from food are likely to have very expensive urine—in other words, they are spending money on supplemental vitamins only to have most of those water-soluble vitamins excreted in their urine. Whether, and how much, vitamin supplementation is needed depends on usual food intake. It is wise to remember that the problems associated with vitamins are at the extremes—excessively low or excessively high intakes.

The Short of It

- Thirteen vitamins are known to be essential, although only small amounts are needed daily.
- Many athletes do not meet recommended intakes because they consume too few calories and vitamin-rich foods.
- The B-complex vitamins do not contain energy, but they are needed for proper energy metabolism.
- Athletes should consume antioxidant-rich diets, which include ample amounts of fruits, vegetables, and whole grains.
- Vitamins can be obtained from foods in which they naturally occur, foods that have been fortified, and vitamin supplements.
- *Caveat emptor*—Buyer beware! Some vitamin supplements may contain high doses.
- The problems are at the extremes—too low or excessive vitamin intake.

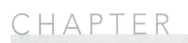
Minerals

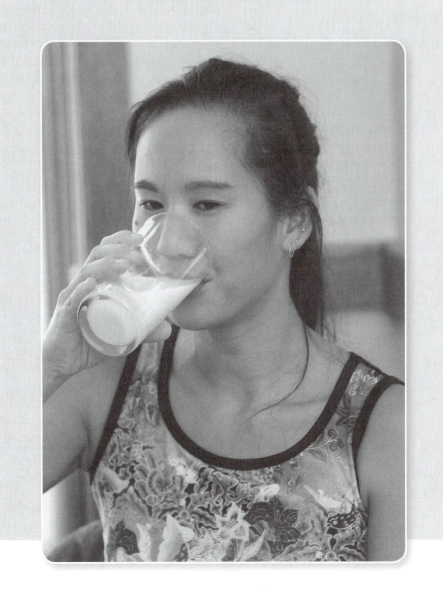

In this chapter, you will learn the following:

✓ The differences between vitamins and minerals
✓ The role of calcium in bone health
✓ The effect of iron deficiency
✓ Foods that are excellent sources of minerals

"Tell me what you eat, and I will tell you what you are."

Jean Anthelme Brillat-Savarin, French lawyer, politician, and gourmet who wrote *The Physiology of Taste* in 1825

The supplement salesman convinced the women's rowing coach that performance would be improved if each rower took a small amount of a liquid mineral supplement each day. The coach bought a bottle and tiny plastic cups and gave the rowers the opportunity to consume some each morning before practice. The rowers didn't care for the taste because it was quite metallic, but they didn't want to disappoint their coach so they dutifully took the tiny cup of elixir each morning. While stretching outside of the boathouse, each rower managed to spill the elixir onto the scruffy grass. When the bottle was empty, the coach thought seriously about ordering more because she perceived that the rowers were improving their performance. She asked the rowers if they thought the elixir was working. "Yes, the grass is greening up nicely," they replied.

What Are Minerals?

Minerals are inorganic compounds that are essential for proper physiological functioning. Along with vitamins, they are referred to as micronutrients because the amounts needed daily are relatively small, measured in milligrams (mg) or micrograms (μg). Twenty-one minerals have been identified as being essential in humans.

Minerals are classified in various ways. One way is based on the amount found in the body. Those that are found in larger amounts are called macrominerals and include calcium, sodium, potassium, and chloride. Those found in smaller amounts are called microminerals, or trace minerals. Examples include iron and zinc.

Another method of classifying minerals is based on function, such as bone formation, red blood cell manufacture, or immune system health support. This chapter focuses on these three major functions. Calcium is highlighted because of its critical role in bone formation. Iron plays a central role in red blood cell formation and the delivery of oxygen. Zinc is one of many minerals needed to support proper immune system function.

Several minerals, including sodium, potassium, and chloride, are electrolytes. Electrolytes have either a positive or a negative charge. Such properties are essential for proper muscle contraction and nerve transmission as well as maintaining fluid balance. Fluid and electrolyte balance is such an important topic for athletes that it will be covered in chapter 9. Although certain minerals are highlighted in this and the next chapter, all minerals play important roles often in combination with vitamins or other minerals.

How Do Minerals Differ From Vitamins?

Like oil and vinegar, vitamins and minerals are often talked about together, but they are more different than they are alike, as shown in table 8.1. Part of the difference is related to their chemical and physiological properties. Compared to water-soluble vitamins, most minerals are not well absorbed, but once absorbed, they are not easily excreted. For example, iron absorption in males is low, typically 2 percent of the iron consumed daily, but iron excretion is also low and not likely to exceed 2 percent daily. Some foods may be a concentrated source of certain vitamins, but minerals in foods tend to be less concentrated. For this reason, daily mineral requirements are best met by eating a variety of foods. For example, if an adult female eats half a cup of cooked spinach, she will receive approximately 70 percent of her vitamin A requirement for the day but only about 10 percent of her iron requirement.

> *A man's health can be judged by which he takes two at a time—pills or stairs.*
>
> **Joan Welsh**, leader of Outward Bound programs, which use wilderness expeditions to build character and inspire self-discovery.

TABLE 8.1   Vitamins and Minerals Compared

	Vitamins	Minerals
Number known to be essential in humans	13	21
Chemical composition	Organic (contain carbon)	Inorganic (do not contain carbon)
Absorption	Generally well absorbed; some competition with each other for absorption	Generally not well absorbed; more competition with each other for absorption
Excretion	Water-soluble vitamins are readily excreted	Most are not readily excreted
Amount found in food	One food may provide nearly all of the amount recommended daily	Generally found in small amounts in food; daily requirement is usually gathered from a variety of foods
Potential for toxicity	Generally large margin of safety between recommended amount and toxic amount	Generally smaller margin of safety between recommended amount and toxic amount

How Do Minerals and Exercise Affect the Body?

Although all of the 21 minerals are important, two are usually emphasized—calcium and iron. These receive the most attention because they are often lacking in the diet, which can lead to well-known deficiency diseases. Zinc also receives attention because of its role in the immune system.

Effect of Minerals on Bones

Eight minerals are involved in bone formation, but two, calcium and phosphorus, make up 80 to 90 percent of the mineral content of bone. Phosphorus is abundant in food and well absorbed, so most discussions of bone mineral content focus on calcium. For proper bone development and maintenance, the nutrient focus is usually calcium and vitamin D. Vitamin D acts as a hormone, which helps to regulate calcium absorption and excretion.

Bone growth requires a sufficient amount of minerals to be present, particularly calcium and phosphorus. Bones lengthen and thicken during childhood and adolescence. This is a critical time for building strong bones. After age 35 calcium is slowly lost from bone. In females, the loss is strongly influenced by the hormone **estrogen**. Bone loss speeds up when estrogen levels are substantially reduced after **menopause**, typically around age 50. However, low estrogen levels can also occur in young female athletes when menstruation is absent or depressed. This condition is known as **athletic amenorrhea** and is detrimental to the athlete's health.

estrogen—One of the female sex hormones.

menopause—The permanent cessation of menstrual activity at around age 50.

athletic amenorrhea—The absence or suppression of menstruation as a result of athletic training.

bone mineral density—The amount of mineral in bone.

cortical bone—Dense, compact bone that forms the surface of the bone.

trabecular bone—Less stiff "spongy" bone that is found at the ends of the bone.

Bone is constantly being remodeled by the cells that dissolve bone, known as osteoclasts, and the cells that form bone, known as osteoblasts. Childhood and adolescence are times when minerals are readily deposited in bones. In young adults the amount of bone dissolved is essentially equal to the amount formed. As people age, the balance shifts and the activity of osteoclasts outpaces that of osteoblasts. One of the natural consequences of aging is a loss of **bone mineral density**. However, the loss can be slowed with proper diet and exercise.

Nearly 80 percent of bone is made up of **cortical bone;** the remaining 20 percent is **trabecular bone**. Trabecular bone is found at the ends of the bones and below the surface, such as in the wrists, spine, femur, and hip. Trabecular bone has a much higher turnover rate than cortical bone, so loss of bone mineral is more likely in trabecular bone. Over time the loss of bone mineral results in bone fragility and a deterioration of the bone's underlying structure. This increases the risk of fractures, especially in the spine, wrist, and hip.

All people should focus on reaching peak bone density and slowing the loss of bone mineral to the extent possible, both of which are affected by exercise and dietary intake. In women, an additional significant factor is estrogen concentration because estrogen affects the number, activity, and life span of the osteoclasts. A decline in estrogen favors the dissolution of bone by allowing osteoclasts to be present in greater numbers, to be more metabolically active, and to live longer than osteoblasts.

If bones are so important, why does the body remove calcium from them? Bone represents a huge storage site of calcium, approximately1 million milligrams, which can be tapped to help maintain blood calcium concentration. Having a stable amount of calcium in the blood ensures that calcium will always be present for cellular activity, especially of nerves and muscles. These tissues cannot function without adequate calcium. Ideally, people should consume an adequate amount of calcium daily; in the absence of adequate calcium intake, the body looks to bone as a source of calcium.

Two mechanisms, both hormonally controlled, occur when dietary intake of calcium is low. When calcium is needed in the blood quickly, it is provided by bone fluid, which surrounds the membranes around bone cells. When calcium is needed over the long term as a result of months and years of low calcium intake, the body draws from the calcium deposited in the bone itself. The calcium typically comes from trabecular bone because it is more metabolically active than cortical bone. A simple analogy is that calcium is deposited in the bone bank while a person is young and withdrawn when needed as the person ages.

Approximately 90 percent of **peak mineral density** in bone is achieved during childhood and adolescence. The remaining 10 percent occurs between ages 20 and 35. The ultimate amount of mineral that can be deposited in bone is genetically determined, but exercise, hormones, and calcium intake are very important factors. Weight-bearing exercise results in mechanical stress on the bone that results in more calcium being put in bones. High-impact activities, such as running and jumping, and sports that include such activities, such as gymnastics, help children and adolescents to build strong bones. Age-appropriate strength training also stresses bone and contributes to peak mineral density.

peak mineral density—Maximum bone density, or the time period in which the bone contains the highest amount of mineral.

In addition to exercise, proper vitamin and mineral intake is needed. Calcium requirements increase during infancy and childhood, reaching their highest levels between ages 9 and 18 when 1,300 milligrams of calcium are needed each day. In addition, 5 micrograms of vitamin D daily is recommended for proper metabolism of calcium and phosphorus. Health and fitness professionals are concerned that many people will not achieve peak bone mineral density because they are sedentary and consume low-calcium diets from a very early age. Some of these individuals will also lack sufficient vitamin D, either due to low vitamin D consumption through food or lack of exposure to UV light. Ultraviolet light helps the body convert a compound in the skin to vitamin D.

After age 35 the emphasis shifts to first preventing and then slowing the loss of bone mineral to the extent possible. The key to preventing or slowing bone loss before the onset of menopause is the intake of calcium via food or supplementation. Adults ages 19 to 50 should consume 1,000 milligrams of calcium and 5 micrograms of vitamin D daily. After age 50 adults should consume 1,300 milligrams of calcium daily. The vitamin D requirement increases substantially to 10 micrograms for those 51 to 70 years old. It increases to 15 micrograms for those over age 70 because they are more likely not to get adequate exposure to sunlight.

⭐ **SUCCESS STORY**

Stella Lucia Volpe, University of Pennsylvania

"Nutrition science and exercise science have always been a natural combination for me. Combining my knowledge in both areas to conduct research in obesity prevention, thyroid hormone function improvement, and osteoporosis prevention has been motivating and challenging. The environmental, applied, and molecular research that is occurring here at Penn, and throughout the world, will help to advance these sciences and result in better health outcomes for our nation and the world."

The preceding quote is from Stella Lucia Volpe, PhD, RD, LDN, FACSM, associate professor and Miriam Stirl Term Endowed Chair, University of Pennsylvania, School of Nursing.

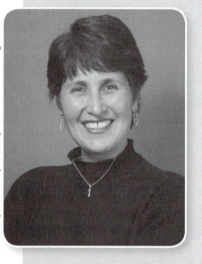

Courtesy of University of Pennsylvania School of Nursing.

"Research is such an exciting part of my career," Stella says. "Each study that I conduct brings new insight for me, both in terms of what the outcomes are and in getting to know participants in the studies, and learn about how the study impacts their lives. I will never forget my chromium study. This study was with overweight, middle-aged women who were given a placebo or a chromium supplement, in a double-blind fashion, and who were also placed on a weightlifting and walking program. As is typical with most of my research, I had a number of graduate and undergraduate students assisting me (to whom I am always grateful!). The participants had to lift weights in the same gym as the university students, and at first, they were a bit embarrassed lifting weights next to very fit, young students. However, after about a month, the neatest thing happened—the participants made friends with students and looked forward to being there with them. I realize this is not focused on the study with chromium supplementation; however, as a researcher, I enjoy human research because I enjoy watching people become more confident in studies like these, in which exercise had not been a part of their lives for a while, or never at all, and then, participants gain a lot of confidence over time. I have seen this in other training studies as well. In addition, the confidence that increases in my graduate and undergraduate students who work on these studies is also a joy to see."

The greatest calcium challenge for women is when estrogen is substantially reduced. For most women this is a result of menopause, which occurs at about age 50. However, it may be the result of athletic amenorrhea at any age. This condition can occur in highly trained female athletes, such as distance runners, who consistently have a low caloric (energy) intake and a high caloric (energy) expenditure from exercise. These women tend to undereat daily. The imbalance between calorie intake and expenditure results in an energy deficit that alters various menstrual hormones including estrogen. Studies have shown that a highly trained female long-distance runner in her mid-20s with long-standing athletic amenorrhea can have the bone density of a 50-year-old woman (Cobb et al., 2003).

Low levels of estrogen speed up the loss of calcium from bone because estrogen's powerful positive influence is lost. Adequate calcium and vitamin D, via diet alone or with supplements, are critical to slow the loss of calcium from bone, but the loss cannot be offset completely by diet or supplementation. Further, adequate calcium intake at this point in life cannot make up for low peak mineral density. The window of opportunity to mineralize bone to its maximum occurs predominantly in childhood and adolescence and to a small degree until age 35. It cannot be achieved later in life.

High-impact exercise may help to maintain bone mineral density in postmenopausal women, but from a practical perspective, many older women are unable or afraid to engage in high-impact, weight-bearing activities. Walking is encouraged to maintain muscle strength and stability, but it does not put enough mechanical stress on the bones to prevent calcium loss. The most practical approach may be a well-planned, supervised resistance training program.

The requirement for calcium is high throughout the life cycle with adult males and females up to age 50 needing 1,000 milligrams of calcium daily. Milk is one of the most concentrated sources, containing approximately 300 milligrams in 8 ounces (240 ml). However, many adults cannot tolerate milk or milk products because they lack a sufficient amount of lactase, the enzyme needed to break down milk sugar (lactose). It is possible to consume enough calcium daily from nondairy sources; however, a variety of calcium-containing foods need to be consumed. For example, 1 ounce of almonds and 3 ounces of clams each contain about 75 milligrams of calcium, but together they contribute only half of the calcium contained in a glass of milk. Dark green, leafy vegetables are also good sources of calcium.

Some foods have substantial amounts of calcium added, such as soy milk, rice milk, and calcium-fortified orange juice, and this calcium is well absorbed. Similarly, calcium supplements provide calcium, which is best absorbed when taken in doses of 400 to 500 milligrams. Vitamin D also increases calcium absorption and is added to milk and to many calcium supplements.

Despite a number of ways to obtain calcium, surveys show that calcium intake is low in at least 50 percent of adult women and 40 percent of adult men. Surveys of athletes generally show a relationship between low caloric intake and low mineral intake, but the amount of calcium consumed varies depending on whether the person consumes dairy products or calcium-fortified foods. In some cases, calcium intake from food is so low that calcium supplementation is the wise thing to do.

Effect of Minerals on Red Blood Cells

Many athletes are involved in sports that depend on aerobic metabolism and optimal oxygen delivery. Oxygen is transported from the lungs to exercising muscle via hemoglobin, an iron-containing protein found in red blood cells. When a hemoglobin molecule is fully saturated with iron, it can carry four molecules of oxygen. Each red blood cell contains more than 250 million molecules of hemoglobin, so it is easy to see why iron is critical to optimal oxygen delivery.

Athletes should have their iron status assessed on a regular basis, and some excellent laboratory tests are available to do so. One of the most common tests shows the amount of hemoglobin in the blood. Another test measures hematocrit, which is the proportion of blood that is red blood cells. When these measures drop below the normal range, then **anemia** is present and oxygen delivery is impaired. A physician can correctly interpret the results of the tests and determine whether iron-deficiency anemia is present. Although iron deficiency is the most common cause of anemia, it is not the only one. One of the symptoms of iron-deficiency anemia is fatigue, which has a negative impact on performance, particularly endurance exercise. However, there are many causes of fatigue including a lack of carbohydrate in the diet. Thus, self-diagnosis of iron-deficiency anemia is never recommended.

anemia—Too few red blood cells or too little hemoglobin in red blood cells.

Iron-deficiency anemia is usually caused by a low intake of dietary iron. It is most prevalent in female athletes who have a high caloric expenditure but low caloric intake, such as long-distance runners and gymnasts, but it can happen to any female athlete. The intake of iron is often low in female endurance athletes, especially those who eliminate red meat and other excellent sources of iron from their diets. Occasionally, iron-deficiency anemia occurs in adolescent male athletes and adult male long-distance runners.

In addition to low iron intake, another contributing factor to iron-deficiency anemia may be iron loss. For females of childbearing age, menstruation is the most common cause of blood loss. Both male and female athletes, particularly distance runners, risk blood loss if they consistently consume medications that result in bleeding, such as aspirin. Although the amount of blood and iron lost this way is much smaller when compared to menstrual losses, the loss can occur daily and over time can be enough to cause iron deficiency.

If blood is lost and if iron intake is low over time, the risk for developing iron-deficiency anemia is increased. Several minerals other than iron are lost when blood is lost, but deficiencies generally appear first for iron because of its critical role in red blood cell formation and the sheer number of red blood cells that must be produced each day.

Once a physician diagnoses iron-deficiency anemia, high-dose iron supplements are prescribed. The dose is high to resupply the iron needed to fully saturate hemoglobin and to build back depleted iron stores in the liver. This typically takes about six months. Self-prescribed iron supplements are not recommended for two reasons: They will not resolve the fatigue if iron deficiency is not the cause, and it is extremely dangerous for some people to take iron supplements because they store too much iron in the liver.

Iron can be found in both animal and plant foods. Animal sources include meat, poultry, and fish, particularly clams and oysters. The iron in animal sources is heme iron, a form that is easily absorbed. Plant foods, such as beans and legumes, are also excellent sources of iron, but the form of iron is nonheme, which is not absorbed as well. Iron can be gathered from a number of plant foods such as green, leafy vegetables and breads and cereals, which have iron added.

Effect of Minerals on the Immune System

Prolonged endurance exercise, rigorous training, and poor dietary intake are known to depress the immune system. Many endurance athletes struggle with repeated upper respiratory tract infections because viruses can establish a toehold during prolonged and rigorous training. From a dietary perspective, a decline in immune cell function occurs as a result of a low intake of protein, some vitamins, and at least two minerals—iron and zinc. Iron deficiency has been previously discussed, so the focus of this section is zinc.

Zinc is a part of at least 100 enzymes, many of which help immune cells to function optimally. Athletes may lose zinc in sweat and urine, especially when strenuously exercising in the heat. Therefore, they must consume an adequate amount daily. Although daily requirements can easily be met by consuming zinc-containing foods, endurance athletes usually do not consume such foods. Studies suggest that up to 90 percent of endurance athletes fall short of the recommended daily intake for zinc because of a low food (caloric) intake, the consumption of a low-protein, high-carbohydrate diet, or the elimination of red meat and milk from their diets (Lukaski, 2000).

The obvious solution would appear to be zinc supplementation, but excess zinc intake depresses the immune system. Thus, athletes need to consume enough, but not too much zinc. For some endurance athletes the best approach would be to increase the intake of red meat and milk, which would provide more zinc, protein, and calories. For others, zinc supplementation would be warranted, but a wise approach would be to limit zinc supplements to no more than 15 milligrams daily. This dose is thought to be safe. Too high a dose of zinc interferes with the absorption of other minerals such as copper.

Zinc is found in protein-containing foods such as meat, poultry, fish, milk, and milk products. As with iron, animal sources of zinc are easily absorbed. Legumes and whole grains are the best plant sources, but absorption from these sources is lower than absorption from animal sources. When grains are processed, zinc is lost, and unlike with iron, there is no law that requires that it be added back. Risk for low zinc intake is associated with a low intake of calories, meat, and milk.

What Is the Recommended Daily Intake of Minerals?

Table 8.2 on page 104 lists the Dietary Reference Intakes (DRIs) for selected minerals for male and nonpregnant female adults between the ages of 19 and 50. The table also lists the tolerable upper intake level (UL), an estimate of the highest level that can be consumed daily that is not likely to cause a health problem. Intakes above the UL can be toxic and are not recommended. Although these recommendations were developed for people who are lightly active, athletes also use these values as a guideline for daily mineral intake.

The table highlights several general issues about minerals. Females need less than, or an equal amount to, males with one notable exception—iron. The daily

TABLE 8.2   Dietary Reference Intakes (DRIs) for Selected Minerals

Mineral	DRI—adult* male	DRI—adult* nonpregnant female	Tolerable upper intake level
Calcium	1,000 mg	1,000 mg	2,500 mg
Phosphorus	700 mg	700 mg	4,000 mg
Magnesium	400 mg (19-30 years); 420 mg (31-50 years)	310 mg (19-30 years); 320 mg (31-50 years)	350 mg (supplement sources only)
Zinc	11 mg	8 mg	40 mg
Iron	8 mg	18 mg	45 mg
Fluoride	4 mg	3 mg	10 mg
Manganese	2.3 mg	1.8 mg	11 mg
Copper	900 μg	900 μg	10,000 μg
Iodine	150 μg	150 μg	1,100 μg
Selenium	55 μg	55 μg	400 μg
Molybdenum	45 μg	45 μg	2,000 μg
Chromium	35 μg	25 μg	Not established
Boron	Not established	Not established	20 mg
Nickel	Not established	Not established	1 mg
Vanadium	Not established	Not established	1.8 mg

*ages 19 to 50

mg = milligram; μg = microgram

Data from: Institute of Medicine, 1997, 2000, 2001.

need for five minerals is very small, measured in micrograms. The DRI or UL has not yet been established for several minerals. In the case of boron, nickel, and vanadium there is enough scientific data to set an upper-level value but not enough evidence to establish the amount needed daily. In other words, we need much more information about minerals.

One of the biggest concerns of athletes is the effect that exercise, particularly rigorous training, might have on mineral requirements. Exercise, especially in hot and humid conditions, can result in profuse and prolonged sweating, and some minerals are lost in sweat. Losses of sodium can be substantial in some athletes. That puts them at risk for fluid and sodium imbalances that can be fatal. This is such an important issue that it is covered extensively in chapter 9. Other minerals that may be lost in sweat include chloride, potassium, iron, calcium, zinc, copper, and magnesium. However, the losses of these minerals are generally small and would likely be covered by the safety margins built into the DRIs.

Which Minerals Are Likely to Be Deficient?

Athletes can obtain adequate amounts of all 21 minerals from food if they choose a variety of mineral-rich foods and consume a sufficient number of calories. However, surveys show that many athletes are deficient in one or more minerals because of poor food choices and inadequate food intake. Calcium, iron, and zinc are three minerals that are often lacking in athletes' diets as a result of lower-than-recommended intakes. Iron and zinc are also considered to be indicators of the other trace minerals. In other words, if dietary iron and zinc intakes are low, consumption of dietary copper, chromium, selenium, and manganese are also likely to be low.

The athletes at greatest risk for low calorie and mineral intakes are those in weight-restricted sports, such as wrestlers and jockeys, and those in low-body-weight sports, such as distance running, female gymnastics, and female ballet dancing. Most minerals are gathered from many different foods because any one food does not typically have a large amount of any mineral. For example, red meat is an excellent source of iron, containing approximately 2 milligrams in 3 ounces (90 g), but this is far short of the daily recommendation of 8 or 18 milligrams, depending on gender and age. However, red meat is just one source of iron. Iron is also found in clams, beans and legumes, green, leafy vegetables, and dried fruits such as raisins, and it is added to foods made from flour such as breads and cereals. Over the course of the day each of these foods contributes to overall iron intake. When athletes restrict their food intake or do not eat a variety of foods, they have a harder time taking in the total amount needed daily.

The two minerals that receive the most attention are calcium and iron. These minerals are often deficient in the diets of both active and sedentary adults, and dietary deficiencies over time can lead to medical conditions. A lack of calcium over decades results in low bone mineral density, known as osteopenia, which increases the risk for **osteoporosis**. A low iron intake can result in iron deficiency that, if not reversed, may progress to iron-deficiency anemia.

osteoporosis—A disease characterized by low bone mineral density and weakened bone structure.

Because calcium and iron are so important and many people do not consume adequate amounts in their diets, it is tempting to see supplemental calcium or iron as a simple solution. Recall that knowing how much calcium and iron you consume in foods is a good indication of how much of the trace minerals are being consumed. Supplementing calcium and iron may solve the problems of deficiencies in these minerals, but will not address other mineral deficiencies, particularly of the trace minerals such as zinc.

How Can Athletes Get the Minerals They Need?

Athletes are likely to get the minerals they need if they do two things: eat enough calories and eat a variety of healthful foods. A healthful diet consists of an adequate number of calories from a variety of foods such as fruits, vegetables, whole-grain breads and cereals, beans and legumes, lean sources of protein, and fat found in nuts, seeds, and oils.

Nutrition Bite

Superfoods!

Most people know that milk is an excellent source of calcium and that red meat is a good source of iron. However, some foods that are mineral superstars are not very well known. The following foods may not get the recognition they deserve because they are not mainstream foods in North America:

- Sardines with bones (3 oz has more calcium than a glass of milk)
- Tofu preserved with calcium (1/2 cup has almost the same amount of calcium as a glass of milk)
- Steamed clams (clams have nine times the amount of iron that red meat does)
- Iron-fortified oatmeal and ready-to-eat breakfast cereals (fortified cereals have three times the amount of iron found in beef)
- Steamed oysters (oysters are extremely high in zinc)

Food choices have a tremendous impact on the amount of minerals consumed. For example, consider two athletes at a food court at a shopping mall. One orders a popular fast-food meal— six pieces of chicken nuggets, large fries, and a large soft drink. The other decides to eat a Mediterranean plate, which consists of hummus, pita bread, lentil pilaf, tabouli (bulgur, tomato, onion, and mint salad) and feta cheese, and a mango smoothie. Table 8.3 shows the difference in mineral intake between the two meals.

The two meals have approximately the same caloric content, but the amount of minerals that each athlete consumes is considerably different. The Mediterranean plate has a much greater variety of foods, and many of them are minimally processed. Foods that are not as refined typically contain more minerals because fewer minerals are lost in processing. The Mediterranean meal also contains grains and legumes, which contribute several minerals. Many typical fast-food meals, such as chicken or a burger with fries and a soft drink, lack fruits and vegetables, foods that contribute small amounts of several minerals.

How Do Food and Supplement Sources of Minerals Compare?

Minerals occur naturally in foods, are added to foods via fortification, and are obtained from supplements. When minerals occur naturally in foods, minimal processing results in a higher mineral content. A good piece of advice is to eat foods that are less processed and more like the original farm-grown product. Table 8.4 compares whole wheat and bleached white flours and illustrates just how many minerals can be lost in the processing. A recommendation for greater mineral intake is to eat whole-grain breads and cereals rather than highly processed grain products.

Consuming all the necessary minerals in the proper quantities from foods in which those minerals naturally occur is possible and desirable. However, people often choose foods that have a lower nutrient content. For example, when white

TABLE 8.3 Mineral Content of Two Meals Compared

MEAL 1: FAST-FOOD CHICKEN MEAL

	Energy (kcal)	Calcium (mg)	Iron (mg)	Zinc (mg)	Magnesium (mg)
Six pieces of chicken nuggets	296	31	1.81	1.24	26
Large fries	540	20	1.44	1.23	57
16 oz (480 ml) cola	195	17	0.72	0.05	5
Total	**1,031**	**68**	**3.97**	**2.52**	**88**

MEAL 2: MEDITERRANEAN PLATE AND SMOOTHIE

	Energy (kcal)	Calcium (mg)	Iron (mg)	Zinc (mg)	Magnesium (mg)
1/2 c hummus	218	60	1.93	1.34	36
1 pita bread	170	10	1.96	0.97	44
1/2 c lentil pilaf	122	17	2.23	0.82	41
1/2 c tabouli	100	15	0.62	0.24	18
1 oz (30 g) feta cheese	74	138	0.18	0.81	5
16 oz (480 ml) mango smoothie	334	67	0.72	0.20	16
Total	**1,018**	**307**	**7.64**	**4.38**	**160**

kcal = kilocalorie; mg= milligram; oz = ounce; g = gram; ml = milliliter; c = cup

bread became available in the United States, it became so popular that many people began to suffer from vitamin and mineral deficiencies. This prompted the government to pass food enrichment laws, which mandated that some of the vitamins and minerals lost in processing, such as some of the B vitamins and iron, be added back. The majority of bread sold in the United States today is still made from white flour, but enrichment has resulted in fewer cases of malnutrition.

At first minerals were added singly to foods in response to widespread deficiencies. For example, iodine was first added to salt in the 1920s as a way to prevent **goiter** and is still added to salt today. The fortification of breakfast cereal began in the 1970s.

goiter—Swelling of the thyroid gland due to a lack of iodine.

TABLE 8.4 Mineral Content of Whole Wheat and Bleached White Flours

	Calcium (mg)	Magnesium (mg)	Zinc (mg)	Selenium (µg)
1/2 c whole wheat flour	20	83	1.76	42
1/2 c white, bleached flour	9	14	0.44	21

mg= milligram; µg = microgram

Today, many foods, such as cereal and energy bars, are highly fortified and contain 12 to 20 added vitamins and minerals. They often contain higher amounts of more minerals than would be naturally found in the ingredients alone. These foods are a hybrid, a cross between a food and a mineral supplement. It is currently unknown how well or poorly the minerals in these foods are absorbed.

> *Can we then conclude that supplementation of that vitamin or mineral improves performance by such and such a percentage as demonstrated in a clinical trial? Not in a "real world setting." Most often funded by manufacturers, these tests produce results that are misleading. Mind you, they are not bending the truth by reporting such gains when their product is taken, but are reporting results not typical for a healthy person who eats a sensible diet.*
>
> **Brendan Brazier**, vegan professional triathlete and winner of the 2003 50K Ultra Marathon National Championship

Mineral supplements are sold singly and in combination with other minerals or vitamins, or both. Many supplements contain 100 percent of the recommended daily intake, and some contain amounts that come close to or exceed the tolerable upper intake level. Some contain chemical forms that have high bioavailability, which means that they are exceptionally well absorbed, used, or retained. Mineral supplements are loosely regulated by the U.S. government, and the manufacturer determines the amount of each mineral contained in the pill or tablet. It is possible to consume a large amount of a mineral via supplementation, although mineral toxicities are rare. Table 8.5 lists some of the advantages and disadvantages of the various mineral sources.

TABLE 8.5   Advantages and Disadvantages of Various Mineral Sources

Mineral source	Advantages	Disadvantages
Naturally occurring in food	• Variety of minerals in each food • Good absorption • Food also provides calories as carbohydrate, protein, or fat	• Must choose foods carefully • Must consume sufficient calories • Popular foods high in sugar, fat, or alcohol tend to be low in minerals
Enriched or fortified food	• Minerals are added to popular foods that are eaten daily • Convenient	• Amount of each mineral absorbed is not known • Not all minerals lost in processing are added back • Too many fortified foods may lead to overconsumption of some minerals
Mineral supplement	• Convenient • Acts as insurance against mineral deficiencies when food intake is poor • Reverses a clinical deficiency (e.g., iron deficiency) • May help to prevent or delay some chronic diseases (e.g., osteoporosis)	• Amount contained may be excessive, which is difficult for consumers to judge • Easy to overconsume one mineral to the detriment of other minerals • May interfere with mineral absorption from food

Nutrition Bite

It is shocking news when a top athlete tests positive for a banned substance. In many cases the athlete denies taking the illegal substance and claims that it must have been in a dietary supplement. The truth will probably never be known because someone taking a banned substance will likely blame it on supplement usage. But some athletes are telling the truth—and paying a big price—because they innocently ingested a contaminated supplement.

It has been well documented that some dietary supplements are contaminated with anabolic steroids. Although the extent of this occurrence is not known, a reasonable estimate is that one in four supplements poses a risk for contamination. Studies have found contaminants in vitamin, mineral, protein, creatine, and herbal supplements that are legally for sale in countries around the world (Maughan, 2005). How did the contaminants get in these supplements? In some cases it was the result of a lack of quality control by the manufacturer, but some may be intentionally contaminated. Most sport governing bodies have zero tolerance for a positive drug test, and athletes are punished even if they had no idea that the supplement contained a banned substance.

Athletes can protect themselves from contaminated supplements by doing the following:

- Keeping supplement use to a minimum
- Choosing supplements that are certified by an independent testing organization such as NSF International
- Buying supplements sold by well-known companies
- Rejecting supplements that sound too good to be true

The Short of It

- Twenty-one minerals are known to be essential.
- Obtaining enough of all essential minerals from food is possible and desirable.
- Many athletes do not consume a sufficient amount of several minerals because their diets are low in calories and lack mineral-rich foods.
- Calcium intake is critical to achieving peak bone mineral density and is a factor in preventing or slowing the loss of calcium from bones.
- Adequate iron intake is important, especially for endurance athletes, because iron-deficiency anemia results in fatigue and reduces endurance capacity.
- Zinc and other minerals are necessary for proper immune system function.
- More foods are being fortified with minerals, and mineral supplements are popular, but the extent to which these minerals are being absorbed is not known.

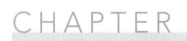

Water, Electrolytes, and Fluid Balance

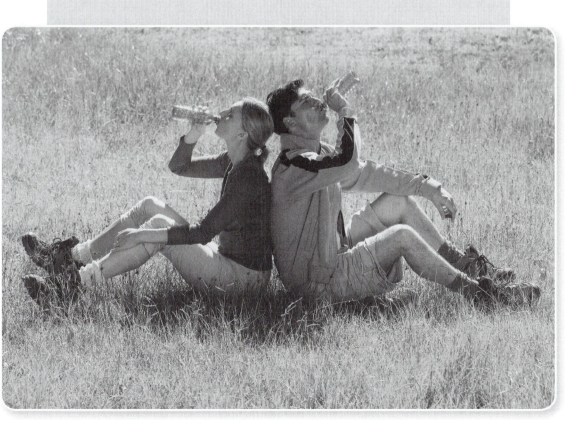

In this chapter, you will learn the following:

✓ Basic facts about water and sodium

✓ Factors that affect water and electrolyte balance in athletes

✓ General guidelines for water and sodium intake before, during, and after exercise

✓ How athletes can determine whether they are dehydrated

> "If there is magic on this planet, it is contained in water."
>
> **Loren Eiseley**, anthropologist and writer (1907-1977)

Some of the most shocking deaths in athletes have been a result of severe water and electrolyte imbalances. Such tragedies include collegiate wrestlers who died when they severely dehydrated themselves in an effort to "cut" weight, a famous bodybuilder who died from cardiac arrest due to potassium depletion, and a 28-year-old woman running the Boston Marathon who developed low blood sodium. In some cases, these athletes voluntarily pushed the envelope too far; in other cases, they made critical mistakes because of lack of knowledge. Although such deaths are rare, they are preventable. Athletes and those who work with them must understand the complex relationships among water, electrolytes, and exercise, especially in the heat.

What Is Homeostasis and How Is It Maintained?

A fundamental principle for the body's survival is **homeostasis**. The word was coined from two Greek words, *homeo*, meaning "the same," and *stasis*, meaning "to stay." To survive, the body must be able to react to changes that threaten its ability "to stay the same." All the body's systems are subject to change, but fluid balance is one of the best examples because of the many changes that can occur as a result of exercise, some of them quite quickly.

homeostasis—The tendency to return to a normal physiologic state.

Depending on the person, 40 to 70 percent of body weight is water; thus, water plays a critical role in maintaining homeostasis. Water is lost from the body in four ways and is supplied in three ways. Water is lost as a result of the following:

■ Ventilation (breathing)

■ Nonsweat skin losses (body water used to keep skin from drying or cracking)

■ Sweat

■ Excretion (primarily in urine)

Water is supplied from the following:

■ Beverages

- Food
- Chemical reactions that produce water

Under nonstressful conditions, such as sitting at room temperature, homeostasis is easy to maintain because water losses are small and water is readily replaced by consuming food and beverages. Balance is largely a result of increasing or decreasing urine output and drinking more or less water in response to thirst.

Exercise, especially in the heat, is a substantial challenge to water homeostasis. Sweating results in a considerable loss of water, and water intake cannot typically keep pace. The body's usual regulatory mechanisms under nonstressful conditions, urine volume and thirst, are simply overwhelmed. Those who exercise at high altitude also lose more water when breathing than they do when exercising at sea level, and this also challenges homeostasis.

How Is Water Distributed in the Body?

For simplicity's sake, body water is categorized as intracellular fluid (ICF) and extracellular fluid (ECF). Intracellular fluid is all the water contained within cells and constitutes approximately two thirds of all the water in the body. Extracellular fluid is all the water outside of cells. It is primarily found in the interstitial fluid, which is the water between the cells, but the water in the blood is also categorized as ECF. Before water can get into cells, it must pass through the extracellular fluid.

What Keeps Water Balanced?

Two major factors involved in water balance are osmosis and electrolytes. Osmosis is the movement of a fluid from a greater concentration to a lesser concentration so that the concentrations will equalize. This would not be an issue if the fluids in the body were just made up of water. However, the fluids inside and outside of the cells contain electrolytes. Electrolytes are particles that carry an electrical charge, either positive or negative. The electrolytes that are critical for fluid balance in the body include sodium (Na^+), potassium (K^+), and chloride (Cl^-), as well as bicarbonate (HCO_3^-) and phosphate (PO_4^{3-}).

Extracellular fluid (i.e., blood and interstitial fluid) is high in sodium and low in potassium, whereas intracellular fluid is high in potassium and low in sodium as shown in figure 9.1. Similarly, ECF contains chloride and bicarbonate, which are negatively charged ions, whereas ICF is high in the negative ion, phosphate. Under normal conditions, water balance is maintained because the total concentration of the charged particles in each fluid compartment is the same.

Exercise challenges the body's ability to maintain water and electrolyte balance. For example, sweating can result in large losses of water from the blood. The loss of water results in a higher concentration of sodium in the blood. In response, water moves from the cells into the blood to reestablish homeostasis. This is but one example of how exercise affects water balance.

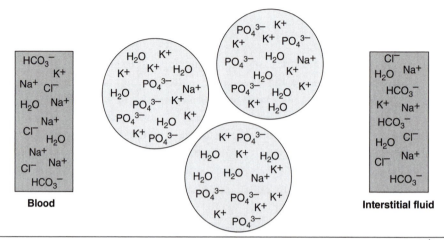

When the body is in fluid balance, most of the water (H_2O), potassium (K^+), and phosphate (PO_4^{3-}) will be in cells and most of the sodium (Na^+), chloride (Cl^-), and bicarbonate (HCO_3^-) will be in the blood.

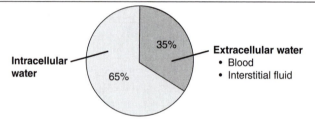

35%

Extracellular water
- Blood
- Interstitial fluid

Intracellular water

65%

FIGURE 9.1 Water and electrolyte balance.

Adapted, by permission, from M. Dunford, 2009, *Exercise nutrition, version 2.0* (Champaign, IL: Human Kinetics), 33.

★ SUCCESS STORY

Bob Murray, Cofounder of Gatorade Sports Science Institute

Ask a sport dietitian about the leaders in the field of fluid and electrolyte balance and undoubtedly the name Bob Murray will be mentioned. As the cofounder and director of the Gatorade Sports Science Institute for over 23 years, and most recently as a private consultant, Dr. Murray has helped expand the knowledge base about how hydration and carbohydrate feeding affect performance.

But his talents do not stop at research. Bob is also adept at translating that scientific knowledge into practical applications. For example, the composition of a beverage affects how fast it is emptied from the stomach and absorbed into the bloodstream. His work in this area helped establish the proper formulations for effective sport drinks. Imagine athletes exercising with thin tubes running down their throats into their stomachs and beyond and you get a rough picture of what that type of research requires! Exercise physiologists, sport nutritionists, certified athletic trainers, coaches, and athletes continue to turn to Dr. Murray for answers to their fluid, electrolyte, and performance questions.

Factors That Affect Water Balance

For most athletes, sweat is the biggest factor in water balance. Exercise results in the production of heat, and the body must respond so that body temperature does not become excessive. Although there are several heat-dissipating methods, one of the most effective is the evaporation of sweat. When sweat evaporates, heat is transported away from the body. Individual sweat rates vary and the environmental temperature is a large influence, but many athletes who exercise in hot conditions will lose 1 to 2 liters of water an hour via sweat. This is the equivalent to a loss of 4 to 8 cups (960-1,920 milliliters) of water per hour. The sidebar "Calculating Sweat Rate" below explains a method for calculating water losses from sweat.

The evaporation of sweat can be hampered by environmental conditions. Exercising in humid conditions is a particular challenge. As the relative humidity increases, the air becomes more saturated with water resulting in reduced evaporation of sweat. The body is still losing water, but sweating is not as effective as a

CALCULATING SWEAT RATE

To determine personal sweat rate, follow these steps:

- Take your body weight nude or in minimal clothing before and after you exercise.
- Measure how much fluid you consume during the exercise.
- Make several measurements under different environmental conditions, such as heat and humidity.
- Enter the appropriate figures into the chart.

A	B	C	D	E	F	G
Preexercise body weight	Immediate[a] postexercise body weight	Change in body weight (A – B)	Fluid consumed during exercise	Sweat loss (C + D)[b]	Exercise time	Personal sweat rate (E/F)
75 kg	73.5 kg	1.5 kg (1,500 g)[c]	480 ml	1,980 ml	60 min	33 ml/min
165 lb	162 lb	3 lb (1,364 g)[d]	2 cups (16 oz) (480 ml)	1,844 ml	60 min	31 ml/min

[a] Do not urinate before taking a scale weight.
[b] 1 g change in weight = 1 ml of fluid
[c] To convert kg to g, multiply by 1,000
[d] To convert lb to g, divide weight in lb by 2.2 and multiply by 1,000
[e] 1 cup = 8 oz; 1 oz = 30 ml

Adapted, by permission, from by R. Murray, 1996, "Calculating sweat rates," *Sports Science Exchange*, 9(63): 6.

sauna suit—Pants and a jacket made of nonbreathable material to facilitate the loss of water weight during exercise.

cutting weight—The process of achieving large and rapid losses of weight, primarily as water, to achieve a particular scale weight before weigh-in.

core temperature—The temperature of the part of the body containing vital organs, such as the heart, liver, and kidneys.

cooling mechanism. Similarly, uniforms and padding can also block the evaporation of sweat. Particularly dangerous is the use of a **sauna suit** by someone who wants to **cut weight** by reducing body water. A sauna suit prevents the evaporation of sweat and causes the athlete to lose water without the benefit of lowering the body's **core temperature**.

Although the loss of sweat while exercising in warm or hot climates receives the most attention, sweating also occurs when exercising in cold temperatures. A particular problem is that the clothing necessary to keep from being too cold at rest or during low-intensity exercise blocks the evaporation of sweat that occurs with higher-intensity exercise. For example, a skier may need to wear a jacket while riding the lift, but the extra clothing blocks the evaporation of sweat while skiing.

There is also evidence that swimmers can lose a substantial amount of water as sweat. For example, one study found that the average sweat rate of elite male water polo players during a match was approximately 750 ml or around 3 cups per hour (Cox, Broad, Riley, & Burke, 2002). Although the rate of water loss is typically lower than that of athletes who exercise on land, the hydration needs of water-sport athletes should not be ignored.

diuretic—A compound that causes an increase in urine output.

For a minority of athletes, another factor affecting water balance is the use of powerful **diuretics**, which quickly and substantially increase the amount of water excreted as urine. Jockeys, wrestlers, and bodybuilders are among those athletes who want to temporarily reduce the amount of water in the body, either in an effort to rapidly reduce scale weight or to improve appearance. In essence, diuretic use overrides one of the body's primary mechanisms for maintaining water balance—the kidneys' regulation of urine volume.

A small number of athletes experiment with the use of glycerol, a compound that acts to temporarily retain water throughout the body. The idea behind glycerol use is that additional water is temporarily stored and available to offset water losses due to sweating. Glycerol supplements are sold as a powder that is mixed with water or a sport beverage. The glycerol is easily absorbed and distributed throughout the body so water is easily retained. Most studies show that glycerol use does result in water retention, but only a handful of studies have shown that glycerol supplementation improves body temperature regulation, maintains blood volume, or improves performance (Nelson & Roberg, 2007). In other words, it should work in theory, but it has only occasionally been shown to work in practice.

Assuming that athletes do not use diuretics, glycerol, or sauna suits, the factor that is likely to have the greatest influence on water balance, especially when exercising in the heat, is sweat rate. That is why there is so much emphasis on the amount of water lost via sweat during exercise.

Factors That Affect Electrolyte Balance

For some athletes, the biggest factor in maintaining electrolyte balance is the loss of a large amount of sodium in sweat. This loss is highly individual because what constitutes normal sodium loss varies considerably. Some athletes lose relatively little sodium when they sweat; others can lose 1 to 2 liters of sweat per hour. These athletes could lose more than 3,000 milligrams of sodium per hour, which is a substantial amount.

Those who sweat heavily and excrete large amounts of sodium in their sweat are sometimes referred to as salty sweaters. **Salt** crystals on skin, shirts, or hats are evidence of substantial sodium loss via sweat. Case studies of football and tennis players who have large and rapid losses of both water and sodium as a result of extreme sweating when exercising in the heat have shown that they are susceptible to **heat cramps**. Heat cramps can result in total body cramping, which is both painful and debilitating. Replacing the sodium that has been lost resolves the heat cramps. Heat cramps are a form of heat illness.

salt—In this context, salt is sodium chloride.

heat cramps—Cramps that occur as a result of a loss of sodium and water when exercising in a hot environment.

Athletes who exercise in warm temperatures for more than two hours, long-distance athletes, and those who train four or more hours daily are also affected by sodium loss in sweat. Sweating continuously for four to eight hours can result in a sizable loss of sodium during training or competition even in those who typically lose a moderate amount of sodium in sweat.

Contrary to popular opinion, the majority of exercise-related muscle cramps are not usually caused by a lack of sodium or a change in the concentration of potassium,

Nutrition Bite

It can be hard to overcome well-established but incorrect information. As a result of new evidence, some of yesterday's advice is no longer true today.

- The old advice was to drink as much as you can. But some athletes drank so much that they diluted the amount of sodium in their blood, and some died because of it. The new advice is to balance water intake with water loss.

- The old advice was to avoid caffeine because it causes dehydration. Caffeine is a mild diuretic so it was assumed that caffeine intake would cause dehydration. The new advice is that caffeine intake up to 300 milligrams daily (about 2 cups of coffee) does not promote dehydration.

- The old advice was that athletes who were going to be exercising in the heat should not use creatine. This was popular advice in 2000, but studies conducted since then do not support creatine restriction by those exercising in the heat. The new advice: If you use creatine supplements, make sure that you are well hydrated.

calcium, and magnesium. Nonetheless, some athletes take mineral supplements to make sure that they have enough of these electrolytes. Although this is common practice, scientific studies have not shown that electrolyte loss and dehydration are the causes of most exercise-related muscle cramping. Although the primary cause is not known, one theory is that the muscle may temporarily lose its ability to relax.

Under normal circumstances, athletes lose only small amounts of potassium in sweat. But athletes can lose a large amount of potassium if they use potassium-depleting diuretics or suffer from eating disorders that include frequent self-induced vomiting. Such practices are rare but can be life threatening.

Chloride and phosphorus, although vitally important for fluid balance, generally get little attention because they are so prevalent in food and are readily absorbed; also, humans are rarely deficient in these electrolytes. Sodium is the electrolyte that receives the most attention, and rightfully so. It is important to keep an eye on potassium and the other electrolytes, although these are easy to obtain in the proper quantities from food, especially a variety of fruits and vegetables.

Is Precise Regulation of Water Necessary?

Under nonstressful conditions, water intake and loss do not need to be precisely regulated. If a person consumes too much water, the body temporarily becomes overhydrated and the **renal** system responds by increasing the volume of urine. Similarly, if a person consumes too little water, the body becomes temporarily underhydrated and the **hypothalamus** responds by increasing the sensation of thirst. Water imbalance under normal conditions is temporary, relatively small in magnitude, and easy to correct.

renal—Related to the kidneys.

hypothalamus—The portion of the brain that regulates body temperature and water balance.

hyponatremia—Low blood sodium concentration.

Exercise, especially in the heat, requires a more precise approach because substantial changes can occur rapidly, may not be easy to correct quickly, and are potentially fatal. First, body temperature will rise as a result of the exercise itself, the environmental conditions, and any clothing or padding that the athlete wears. Second, water losses may be so substantial that they cannot be offset by water intake during the exercise. Third, sodium may be affected if the duration of the exercise is long, water is overconsumed, and the blood sodium level drops rapidly. This condition is known as **hyponatremia** and can be fatal. For all these reasons, athletes need to regulate their water intake as precisely as they can.

Precise regulation of water intake during exercise can be difficult because of problems associated with intake and absorption. Most athletes do not feel thirsty early in the exercise period even though they are losing a large amount of body water. Gastrointestinal (GI) upset can occur with fluid intake during exercise, which limits the amount the athlete voluntarily consumes. The amount of fluid absorbed from the GI tract during exercise may be less than the amount of water lost in sweat, especially when performing high-intensity exercise in the heat. For all these reasons, it may not be possible for the athlete to replace the water he is losing during exercise (see Why Fluid Balance During Exercise Is a Challenge on page 119).

WHY FLUID BALANCE DURING EXERCISE IS A CHALLENGE

Athletes lose water for the following reasons:

- Body temperature is rising during exercise.
- The environmental temperature is warm or hot.
- Humidity is high.
- Clothing or pads are required.

Athletes don't replace water for the following reasons:

- They don't feel thirsty.
- Opportunities to drink are limited.
- Drinking too much causes nausea.

Why Do Athletes Need Individualized Plans for Fluid and Electrolyte Intake?

Each athlete needs an individualized plan because it is not possible to make a single recommendation about fluid or electrolyte intake for all athletes. The plan needs to focus on water and electrolyte intake before, during, and after exercise. Intake during exercise typically gets the most attention because losses are usually largest during exercise and those losses must be offset as soon as possible. However, the plan will be incomplete if the focus is only during exercise. Athletes should rehydrate completely in the hours after exercise and be well hydrated before the next exercise bout. As a practical issue, the plan must also consider the need for carbohydrate before, during, and after exercise because carbohydrate is often consumed in liquid form.

A basic plan is needed for the athlete's usual training conditions. This plan must account for the fundamental factors that affect fluid balance (see the sidebar Differences Among Water, Fluids, and Sport Beverages on p. 120). That plan must be modified to reflect factors that the athlete may face during competition such as warmer temperatures, greater relative humidity, and GI distress associated with nerves before or during a race or game. Each athlete needs a well-thought-out plan, but that plan must be flexible to match changing conditions. Trial and error is needed to fine-tune the plan.

What Type and How Much Fluid Should Be Consumed?

Athletes must determine the amount and type of fluid that is best to consume given their sport and their individual tolerances and preferences. Typically, athletes make decisions about fluid intake based on three time frames—before, during, and after

DIFFERENCES AMONG WATER, FLUIDS, AND SPORT BEVERAGES

Water and *fluid* are terms that are often used interchangeably, which can be confusing when discussing water and electrolyte balance. Water is H_2O, but anything that is liquid can be a fluid. Fluids are mostly water, but they also contain other compounds. For example, sport beverages may contain electrolytes (such as sodium and potassium), carbohydrate, and caffeine. Each of these compounds has an influence on water or electrolyte balance. In some cases the most appropriate beverage is water, but in other cases a sport beverage is the best choice. When choosing the most appropriate beverage(s) always consider these factors:

■ Intensity and duration of the exercise
■ Environmental conditions, such as the heat and humidity
■ Timing of intake, such as before, during, or after exercise
■ Nutrient composition of the beverage
■ Gastrointestinal tolerance
■ Individual preferences

exercise. The following sections offer general guidelines for each of these periods. These guidelines are good starting points; however, they must be tailored to the individual athlete.

Before Exercise

The type and amount of fluid consumed before exercise depend on the athlete's goals and tolerances. Following are typical goals before exercise:

■ Being fully hydrated
■ Catching up to the extent possible if not fully hydrated
■ Avoiding gastrointestinal upset
■ Consuming carbohydrate, if needed

In its 2007 position stand, the American College of Sports Medicine (ACSM) recommended that athletes consume approximately 5 to 7 milliliters of fluid per kilogram of body weight (ml/kg) in the four hours before exercise. For example, a 220-pound (100 kg) athlete should slowly consume around 500 to 700 milliliters (around 2 or 3 cups) of fluid in the hours before exercise. This amount of fluid will help maintain hydration status, which is assumed to be adequate before exercise, and will typically not cause GI distress. The practical problem with any substantial amount of fluid intake before exercise is urination and the discomfort of having a full bladder during competition or training.

Many athletes do not begin exercise in a well-hydrated state. In such cases the ACSM recommends that an additional 3 to 5 ml/kg be consumed at least two hours before the onset of exercise. Using the same example, a 220-pound (100 kg) athlete who is dehydrated before exercise begins should take in an additional 300 to 500 milliliters (around 1 1/4 to 2 cups) of fluid. In other words, this athlete would want to drink a total of 800 to 1,200 milliliters (3 ¼ to 5 cups) of fluid before exercise. He should begin four hours before exercise and continue drinking as close to the time of the exercise as possible. He will need to determine the actual amount he can tolerate through trial and error.

> *My biggest weakness as an endurance athlete has been in not drinking enough water after training, thereby racing sometimes while dehydrated.*
>
> **Bill Rodgers**, endurance athlete

The choice of fluid before exercise usually is water or a sport beverage with a small amount of carbohydrate. If an athlete is well hydrated, has adequate muscle glycogen stores, and will eat a carbohydrate-containing preexercise meal, then water will be sufficient. For athletes with low muscle glycogen stores, little time to consume food before exercise, or a preference for a sweet-tasting beverage, a sport beverage would be a good choice. To avoid GI upset and promote absorption, this beverage should contain approximately 6 to 8 percent carbohydrate, or 14 to 16 grams of carbohydrate in 8 ounces (240 ml) of water.

Some athletes also consume caffeinated coffee or tea with a preexercise meal. One benefit is that caffeine is a stimulant and can increase awareness. However, too much caffeine before exercise can cause overstimulation of the nervous system, GI upset, and subsequent urination. Thus, athletes need to determine preexercise caffeine tolerance via trial and error. Table 9.1 lists the nutrient composition of various beverages typically consumed by athletes before exercise. Note that the nutrient information is based on an 8-ounce (240 ml) serving, but sport beverages are generally sold in larger containers.

During Exercise

Typical goals for athletes who can consume fluid during exercise are as follows:

- Replacing lost body water
- Avoiding the overconsumption of water
- Replacing sodium, if losses are large
- Avoiding gastrointestinal upset
- Consuming carbohydrate, if needed

In the past, experts often recommended that endurance athletes consume 6 to 12 ounces (180 to 360 ml) of fluid every 15 to 20 minutes during exercise. Such definitive recommendations are no longer made because of the risks associated with

TABLE 9.1 Composition of Various Preexercise Beverages

Product (8 oz or 240 ml)	NON-H$_2$O COMPONENTS							
	Sodium (mg)	Potassium (mg)	CHO (g)	CHO (%)	Caffeine (mg)	Other	Energy (kcal)
Water	trace	trace	0	0	0		0
Black coffee	trace	trace	0	0	~100-200		0
Decaf coffee (black)	trace	trace	0	0	3-12		0
Tea (plain)	trace	trace	0	0	~40-120	Some antioxidants	0
Decaf tea (plain)	trace	trace	0	0	5	Some antioxidants	0
Gatorade G2	160	45	10	4	0		40
Gatorade Thirst Quencher	110	30	14	6	0		50
Gatorade Endurance Formula	200	90	14	6	0	6 mg Ca; 3 mg Mg	50
Gatorade Tiger	135	40	14	6	0		50
Hydrade	91	77	10	4	0	Contains glycerol	55
All Sport Body Quencher	55	50	16	6.5	0		60
Powerade	53	30	19	8	0	May contain B vitamins	72
Accelerade	120	15	15	6	0	4 g protein; 20 mg Ca; 5 mg vitamin E	80

oz = ounce; ml = milliliter; H$_2$O = water; mg = milligram; CHO = carbohydrate; g = gram; kcal = kilocalorie; Ca = calcium; Mg = magnesium the overconsumption of water. Thus, the 2007 ACSM recommendations are for an individualized plan that takes into account environmental conditions, particularly heat and humidity; exercise duration; body size; sweat rate; and loss of sodium and other electrolytes.

For example, a 280-pound (127 kg) American football player in uniform in a warm and humid climate who sweats heavily may need the same amount of fluid during exercise as a 150-pound (68 kg) marathon runner in a hot climate. A male soccer player who sweats heavily will likely lose more water during a rigorous training session than a woman who sweats very little will lose during a 10-kilometer run. To obtain a ballpark figure for water loss during exercise, an athlete should take a scale weight immediately before and immediately after exercise. One liter of water weighs approximately 1 kilogram, or 2.2 pounds. Thus, each pound (0.5 kg) loss of scale weight after exercise represents approximately 2 cups (480 ml) of water lost. This rough estimate can help an athlete establish a working guideline for fluid intake during exercise, which then can be fine-tuned.

For example, an athlete who weighed 2 pounds (1 kg) less after exercise in high heat and humidity could assume that this is the usual amount she will lose under these environmental conditions. The next day the athlete could try to take in approximately 4 cups (1 L) of fluid during exercise. Then she should check her scale weight again. If her weight after exercise is below her weight before exercise, then the 4 cups may not have been enough to restore all the fluid she lost. The next day she could experiment with drinking 4 1/2 cups of fluid during exercise. Or she may be able to restore her scale weight with 3 1/2 cups of fluid. Because each athlete is unique, the general guidelines must be fine-tuned.

In addition to fluid, those engaged in long-distance endurance sports may need to consume sodium during exercise. Athletes in sports such as marathons, triathlons, and ultradistance cycling and running are at risk for losing a large amount of sodium as a result of prolonged sweating. It is not necessary to replace all the sodium lost during exercise at the time of exercise, but it is wise for these athletes to consume some sodium in beverages or foods during exercise to prevent hyponatremia (see the sidebar Hyponatremia on p. 125). Sodium intake also helps the body to maintain its desire to drink; thus, some sodium during endurance exercise may help athletes in these sports to meet their water intake goals.

In addition to long-distance endurance athletes, any athlete who is a salty sweater should have a plan for sodium consumption. This plan may include consuming beverages containing 200 milligrams of sodium in 8 ounces (240 ml). However, those who lose very large amounts of sodium may need a more concentrated source, such as a salt tablet. Products such as Lava Salts and Succeed! contain approximately 340 milligrams of sodium per tablet. The manufacturers caution against using more than two tablets per hour and emphasize that each tablet should be taken with 12 to 16 ounces (360 to 480 ml) of fluid. Most athletes do not need to take salt tablets during exercise.

Some athletes may benefit from consuming carbohydrate during exercise. A common recommendation is 30 to 60 grams of carbohydrate an hour, which provides a source of glucose to exercising muscle and helps to stabilize blood glucose

TABLE 9.2   Composition of Various Beverages Consumed During Exercise

Product (8 oz or 240 ml)	NON-H$_2$O COMPONENTS						
	Sodium (mg)	Potassium (mg)	CHO (mg)	CHO (%)	Caffeine (mg)	Energy (kcal)
Gatorade G2	160	45	10	4	0	40
Gatorade Thirst Quencher	110	30	14	6	0	50
Gatorade Endurance Formula	200	90	14	6	0	50
Gatorade Tiger	135	40	14	6	0	50
All Sport Body Quencher	55	50	16	6.5	0	60
Powerade	53	30	19	8	0	72
Accelerade	120	15	15	6	0	80
1 packet GU, a carbohydrate gel (consumed with water)	40	35	25	N/A	0, 20 or 40	100

oz = ounce; ml = milliliter; H$_2$O = water; mg = milligram; CHO = carbohydrate; kcal = kilocalorie; N/A = not applicable level. This amount of carbohydrate typically is well absorbed and does not result in GI upset. It is convenient to consume carbohydrate in liquid form, but it is equally effective for the carbohydrate to be in the form of a gel, such as GU, or a carbohydrate-containing food, such as a banana. Table 9.2 lists the nutrient composition of various beverages that athletes may consume during exercise.

Most of the research studies of fluid intake during exercise are conducted in endurance athletes. However, fluid intake during exercise is also a concern for athletes in stop-and-go sports, such as soccer and basketball, and those that engage in low-intensity exercise for several hours, such as baseball players and golfers. Well-trained stop-and-go athletes often follow the same fluid and carbohydrate guidelines as endurance athletes because they sweat heavily and also benefit from a small amount of carbohydrate during time-outs or substitutions. However, a baseball player will lose little fluid sitting in the bullpen or dugout during night games in mild temperatures. His fluid needs can be met with water. In fact, some baseball players may find sport beverages to be more detrimental than advantageous because they contribute additional calories and may hamper efforts to lose body fat. This underscores an important point—each athlete needs an individualized plan because each athlete's goals and tolerances are unique.

> **mmol/L**—Millimole per liter; used to measure the amount of a substance, such as an electrolyte in the blood.

HYPONATREMIA

Hyponatremia is the medical term for low blood sodium. Normal blood sodium concentration is 140 **mmol/L**. A blood sodium concentration less than 135 mmol/L is considered low. Exercise-induced hyponatremia is typically defined as a rapid drop in blood sodium to less than 130 mmol/L and is a medical emergency when the concentration is below 125 mmol/L. Such a level is life threatening.

Hyponatremia causes water in the blood to move by osmosis into the cells, which results in the swelling of cells. This is particularly disruptive to nerve cells, and dizziness, confusion, and coma can result. Unfortunately, some endurance athletes have died of hyponatremia.

Hyponatremia is relatively rare; it is most often seen in slow marathon runners, ultraendurance runners, and triathletes. The causes are still under investigation, but it is likely a result of overconsumption of water or other low sodium fluids during exercise and the loss of sodium in sweat (Noakes et al., 2005). Prevention of hyponatremia includes avoiding overconsumption of water, matching water intake with water loss, and consuming sodium during endurance exercise by drinking sodium-containing beverages or eating a salty food, such as salted crackers.

After Exercise

The recovery period begins immediately after exercise. Many athletes train or compete on a near daily basis, so timing is critical for full restoration of lost body water before the next exercise session. Rehydration should be a primary focus after

> *I want to say that those people drinking all that water can get sick and die from water intoxication.*
>
> **A caller**, who said she was a nurse, to a radio station sponsoring a contest to see who could drink the most water without going to the bathroom. One of the contestants died.

exercise. Beverages are a convenient form by which athletes consume some of the carbohydrate, protein, and electrolytes needed for full recovery. Postexercise goals typically include the following:

- Replacing lost body water
- Returning to an adequately hydrated state
- Replacing sodium and other electrolytes that were lost
- Avoiding gastrointestinal upset
- Consuming enough carbohydrate to fully restore muscle glycogen
- Consuming some protein to build and repair muscles

If dehydration has been mild, a normal intake of food and beverages will likely restore hydration status because both fluid and electrolytes will be consumed. However, some athletes experience significant dehydration and they need to rapidly and completely restore the lost fluid. The ACSM recommends that such athletes consume approximately 1.5 liters (50 oz or 6 1/4 cups) of fluid per kg of body weight lost, as measured by comparing pre- and postexercise scale weights. For example, an athlete who loses 3 pounds (1.4 kg) of body weight, will need approximately 2,100 milliliters (70 ounces or 8 3/4 cups) of fluid for rehydration.

Fluid intake after exercise should begin as soon as possible. The amount consumed at any one time will depend on GI tolerance, so full rehydration may take many hours. Water is an appropriate postexercise beverage for restoring body water, but many athletes consume beverages that contain other nutrients that they need, such as carbohydrate and protein. Specially formulated recovery beverages kill two birds with one stone.

The amount of sodium to consume depends on the amount lost in sweat. As a general rule, athletes often consume a beverage with some sodium or lightly salt their food after exercise. Those who have lost large amounts of sodium in sweat typically are more diligent about consuming salt by heavily salting their food or eating foods that are high in sodium, such as pretzels dipped in salt. Under normal conditions, an excessive but temporary sodium intake is not likely to cause a health problem because the kidneys excrete the excessive sodium in the urine.

Other electrolytes that are lost in sweat—calcium, magnesium, or copper—are typically restored by eating nutritious foods such as green, leafy vegetables, fruits, whole-grain breads and cereals, nonfat milk, and calcium-fortified nondairy products such as soy milk. Table 9.3 lists the nutrient composition of some popular beverages that may be consumed after exercise. The amount and composition of beverages needed to restore the water and electrolytes lost will vary according to the person.

TABLE 9.3 Composition of Various Postexercise Beverages

Product	NON-H$_2$O COMPONENTS							
	Sodium (mg)	Potassium (mg)	CHO (g)	Protein (g)	Fat (g)	Caffeine (mg)	Other	Energy (kcal)
Gatorade Protein Recovery Shake (1 can)	260	480	45	20	1.5	0	450 mg Ca	270
Gatorade Energy Drink (12 oz or 360 ml)	200	105	78	0	0	0	8 vitamins	310
Low-fat chocolate milk (8 oz or 240 ml)	153	425	26	8	3	0	288 mg Ca; Other vitamins & minerals	170
High-protein Boost (8 oz or 240 ml)	170	380	33	15	6	0	21 vitamins & minerals	240
Boost (8 oz or 240 ml)	130	400	41	10	4	0	26 vitamins & minerals	240

H$_2$O = water; mg = milligram; CHO = carbohydrate; g = gram; kcal = kilocalorie; Ca = calcium; oz = ounce; ml = milliliter

How Does Dehydration Affect Training, Performance, and Health?

At any time an athlete's hydration status falls on a continuum from low body water to proper hydration to excessive body water, as shown in figure 9.2. The goal is to begin training sessions and competition in a state of proper hydration. Dehydration is the process of losing body water and is typically defined as a loss of 2 percent or more of body weight as water. Dehydration can affect the athlete's ability to perform and to regulate body temperature.

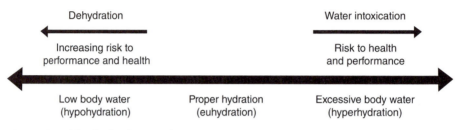

FIGURE 9.2   The hydration continuum.

The majority of hydration research has been conducted with athletes performing endurance or stop-and-go activity in warm, hot, and/or humid environments. For these athletes, the studies show a decline in performance as summarized in table 9.4. Studies also suggest that the greater the degree of dehydration, the greater the degree of performance decline. Thus, it is wise for endurance and stop-and-go athletes who are training and competing in the heat to offset dehydration to the extent possible.

TABLE 9.4   Effects of Dehydration on Aerobic Performance

Sport	Degree of dehydration*	Effect on performance
Basketball	2%	Movement slows, shooting is less accurate, and attention declines. Performance continues to decline as the degree of dehydration increases.
Distance cycling	2.5%	On a 2-hour ride with hills, power output for hill climbing declines.
1,500 m run	2%	Running time increases by 3%.
5,000 or 10,000 m run	2%	Running time increases by 5%.
Soccer	1.5-2%	Playing ability and fitness declines; perceived exertion increases.

* % loss of body weight as water

Data from Armstrong, Costill, Fink, 1985; Baker, Conroy, Kenney, 2007; Baker, Dougherty, Chow, et al., 2007; Ebert, Martin, Bullock, et al., 2007; Edwards, Mann, Marfell-Jones, et al., 2007.

Fewer hydration studies have been conducted in predominantly strength and power athletes, and the ones that have usually involve wrestlers. These studies have generally concluded that a loss of 3 to 5 percent of body weight as water does not affect muscle strength or performance (ACSM, 2007b). However, such a loss does affect the regulation of body temperature, and the risk for elevated body temperature should not be overlooked because it is a potentially fatal condition. Some wrestlers have died in the training room from **hyperthermia** as a result of large and rapid loses of body water when they were already in a dehydrated state.

Normal body temperature is approximately 98.6 °F (37 °C), and 113 °F (45 °C) is incompatible with life. A body temperature elevated above normal increases the risk for **heat illness**, including **heatstroke**. With heatstroke, the athlete's internal temperature is greater than 104 °F (40 °C). Such an elevated temperature negatively affects the function of all the major organs.

> **hyperthermia**—Elevated body temperature.
>
> **heat illness**—A general term for medical symptoms resulting from exposure to heat.
>
> **heatstroke**—A severe form of heat illness that results from an abnormally high body temperature; may be fatal.

The primary risk factors for heatstroke are strenuous exercise in hot and humid conditions, poor physical conditioning, and a lack of acclimatization to the heat. A handful of professional athletes have died in training camp from heatstroke. Because dehydration is often a factor in heatstroke, athletes should minimize dehydration to the extent possible. However, some athletes who experience heatstroke are not dehydrated. In other words, well-trained, well-acclimatized, lean athletes may also experience heatstroke.

Nutrition Bite

Rhabdomyolysis is the rapid breakdown of muscle due to injury. When the muscle cells are damaged, compounds normally found inside the cells are released into the blood. One example is myoglobin, an iron-containing protein found in muscles. Large amounts of myoglobin released into the bloodstream can harm the kidneys.

Athletes sometimes refer to this condition as "rhabdo." It is most common when athletes repeat new exercises to excess. For example, a novice martial artist may practice a kick move to excess, or a new police or military recruit may do hundreds of push-ups. When many muscle cells are damaged, the myoglobin spills over into the urine making the urine the color of tea or cola. This is a warning sign to seek immediate medical attention.

Other examples of athletes who have experienced rhabdomyolysis include bodybuilders, first-time marathon runners, and rugby players who perform an excessive number of squat jumps. Dehydration makes this condition worse, which is another reason that athletes need to be well hydrated before, during, and after exercise.

Signs of Dehydration

There are several relatively simple methods athletes can use on a daily basis to monitor hydration status. These assessments should be conducted immediately after waking.

- **Urine concentration**. Inexpensive urine testing strips can measure urine concentration. Dehydration is associated with a urine specific gravity greater than 1.020.

- **Urine color**. A darker urine color indicates that the athlete is dehydrated. Use of a urine color chart helps to reduce bias and misinterpretation. However, athletes can also use the eyeball test. If urine looks like the color of apple juice, then dehydration is likely. The athlete's urine should appear clear or the color of lemonade. It is important to note that some dietary supplements can darken the color of urine.

- **Scale weight**. A lower scale weight when compared to the previous morning indicates that the athlete is dehydrated. Weight must be taken under the same conditions each day.

- **Thirst**. Thirst typically indicates that the athlete is at least 2 percent dehydrated.

The Short of It

- Water and electrolyte balance is critical for health and performance.
- The evaporation of sweat is a primary way for the body to cool itself.
- Sweating typically represents the largest loss of water during exercise.
- Athletes need to match their fluid loss with their fluid intake.
- Some athletes lose a large amount of sodium during exercise.
- Each athlete needs an individualized plan for fluid and sodium intake before, during, and after exercise.
- Salting food after exercise is one way of replenishing the sodium lost during exercise.
- Simple measures such as scale weight and urine color can help athletes determine whether they are dehydrated.
- Distance athletes need to make sure they do not overconsume water, which can lead to low blood sodium.

CHAPTER 10

Weight, Body Composition, and Performance

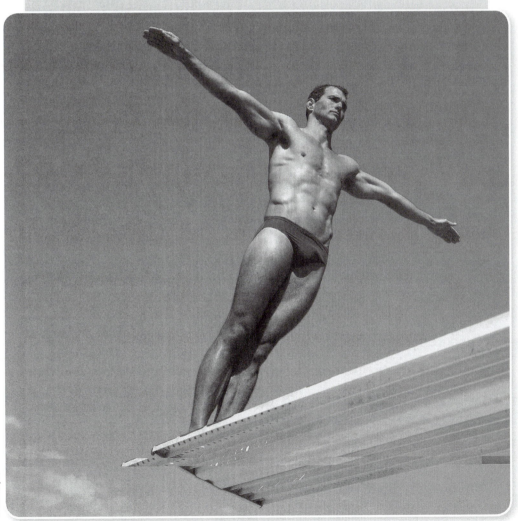

In this chapter, you will learn the following:

✓ General information about body weight and body composition
✓ Methods for determining body composition and their accuracy
✓ How weight and body composition relate to performance
✓ Amount of additional calories and protein needed daily to support muscle growth

"When I'm not in training, I'll walk around the streets at 153 [pounds], but it's not solid; it's my socializing weight."

Sugar Ray Leonard, professional boxer who was named Fighter of the Decade for the 1980s

It's a pretty typical story—a skinny kid wants to become a star athlete. He lives and breathes his sport and practices endlessly, but his body just won't cooperate when it comes to gaining more muscle. He grows taller but can't seem to add a lot of meat to his bones. His father tells him to be patient, because the same thing happened to him when he was growing up. Finally, in his late 20s he begins an intensive resistance training program and his body begins to transform into a lean machine. Everyone marvels at his now-sculpted body and the well-developed muscles bursting out from under his shirt sleeves. Who would have thought that this time-honored tale is also the story of the number one golfer in the world, Tiger Woods? He changed his weight and body composition in a never-ending quest to improve his performance.

What Is Body Weight?

Body weight is a measurement of the total amount of material, known as mass, in the body. It is easily measured in pounds (lb) or kilograms (kg), but this single number gives no indication of the amount of fat, skeletal muscle, bone, or fluid present. Measurements of body composition have been developed to better distinguish among these components.

Measurement of Body Weight

A balance beam or digital scale that has been calibrated is the most accurate measurement of body weight. Home scales are less accurate but widely used because they are convenient. An accurate scale weight is vitally important for athletes whose weight must be certified before competition such as wrestlers, boxers, some martial artists, jockeys, and lightweight rowers. However, because most athletes are personally tracking their weight over time, the important issue is that they repeatedly measure their weight on the same scale.

Body weight is useful information for athletes as long as it is interpreted correctly. One of the best uses of scale weight is to compare weight before and after exercise to determine the amount of fluid lost during exercise (see chapter 9). Athletes who use this as a hydration-tracking method usually measure scale weight on a near-daily basis. They step on a scale before exercise and step on the same scale afterward. Some athletes record the difference in these two weights in a journal.

Comparing scale weight over many months is a way to track large changes in body composition. For example, an American football player whose goal is to increase total body weight by 30 pounds (13.5 kg) primarily by increasing skeletal muscle, can track weight over many months to see if he is progressing toward his goal. Those looking to reduce body weight may also benefit from month-to-month tracking of scale weight. These athletes often take a weight on the same day of the month and write the result on a calendar. It is important to use the same scale each time.

However, scale weight can easily be misinterpreted. Tracking day-to-day weight as a way to determine fat loss is inappropriate because losses in body fat occur slowly. Daily changes reflect changes in water content rather than in body fat. Similarly, a gain in body weight simply indicates that body mass is greater. Returning to the preceding example, a 30-pound weight gain could be an increase in skeletal muscle, body fat, or water. Weight alone does not tell the athlete whether he has met his intended goal—in this case, an increase in skeletal muscle. Those with a distorted body image can misinterpret weight and become too focused on a number that they believe they should not exceed. Lean and muscular athletes may have a high body weight, which may lead some people to think that they are too fat. For these reasons, body composition measurements are needed for correctly interpreting the meaning of changes in scale weight.

> *Right now I'm 185 [pounds], which is really good for me yet very hard for me to maintain. My weight seems high for the average woman, but I've got big bones and I'm maintaining muscle.*
>
> **Lisa Leslie**, former professional American women's basketball player and four-time Olympic gold medalist

Relationship of Body Weight and Fat to Health

There is much emphasis on overweight and obesity and their relationship to health. The tool that is most often used to screen the general population for weight-related health problems is body mass index (BMI). BMI assumes that adult height is stable and that a high BMI is a reflection of excessive body fat. BMI can be determined by using an online calculator (www.cdc.gov/nccdphp/dnpa/bmi).

In general, the risk of dying from **chronic** diseases, such as heart disease and diabetes, increases when BMI falls outside the normal weight category. Not surprisingly, the risk for chronic disease rises as BMI increases and a person becomes overweight or obese. However, this risk is very much influenced by cardiovascular fitness. In other words, two people may be classified as overweight according to

chronic—Lasting over a long period of time.

BMI, but the one who is fit has less risk than the one who is not. What surprises most people is that risk also increases as BMI declines below the healthy weight range. These relationships are shown in figure 10.1.

BMI is not an appropriate health-screening tool to use with athletes. Because of the weight of a large amount of skeletal muscle, a highly muscular athlete with a low percentage of body fat can easily be placed in the overweight or obese category on the BMI chart. One health-screening tool that is used with athletes, as well as the general population, is the measurement of abdominal fat.

The distribution of excess body fat is actually more predictive of health problems than the total amount of body fat. There is a much higher disease risk associated with excess abdominal fat, which is located deep inside the abdominal cavity, than with excessive **subcutaneous fat**. Abdominal fat is also called truncal fat or visceral fat. This type of fat is readily released into the blood, which increases disease risk. Abdominal fat is easily measured by taking a waist **circumference**. If the waist is greater than 40 inches (102 cm) in a man or greater than 35 inches (88 cm) in a woman, then the risk for disease is greater. In addition to waist circumference, other good measures for determining disease risk are blood pressure, blood glucose, and **blood lipids**, such as cholesterol.

subcutaneous fat—Fat located directly under the skin.

circumference—Distance around.

blood lipids—Fats in the blood.

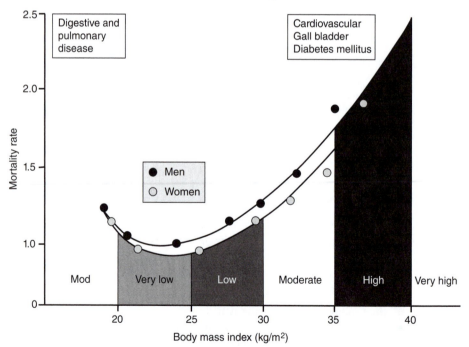

All cause mortality

FIGURE 10.1 The relationship between weight and mortality.

What Is Body Composition?

Simply stated, the body is composed of fat and fat-free tissues. Fat includes essential fat, which is found in many cells and tissues of the body; visceral fat, which surrounds organs; and subcutaneous fat, which is stored under the skin. Typically, the largest amount of fat is found subcutaneously. Fat-free mass (FFM) includes skeletal muscle; nonskeletal muscle, such as the heart; bone; fluids; and organs. The term *lean body mass* is often used interchangeably with *fat-free mass,* but this is incorrect because lean body mass includes FFM and essential fat. Many athletes use the term *lean mass* to refer to skeletal muscle, but skeletal muscle is only one aspect of lean body mass.

Outside of research settings, a two-component model is typically used to determine body composition. In other words, the body is simply divided into fat and fat-free tissues. Using such a simple way to categorize the body introduces error into the process of measuring body composition. For example, bone does not have the same density as muscle, but both bone and muscle are put in the same category.

Accuracy of Body Composition Measurements

The only accurate way to measure body composition directly would be to remove a person's entire body fat and place it on a scale. Obviously, this cannot be done if that person is alive. Thus, all body composition measurements are indirect. The problem with indirect measurements is that they are based on prediction, and there is always error associated with prediction equations.

The amount of error depends on the method used to measure body composition. Even the most precise methods used in research settings have some error, known as the standard error of the estimate (SEE). For example, dual-energy X-ray absorptiometry (DXA, or DEXA) has an error margin of approximately 1.8 percent. This means that if the body is determined to be 13 percent body fat, the actual percentage of body fat is somewhere between 11.2 and 14.8 percent. This range, however, is accurate for only 67 percent of the people who are estimated to be 13 percent body fat. The remaining 33 percent have a percentage of body fat that is below 11.2 percent or above 14.8 percent. This example illustrates the extent of the potential error when estimating body composition.

The inherent errors found in all measurement methods can be compounded by mistakes made by the technician or subject. For example, skinfold measurements require that the technician be well trained in measurement technique. A poorly trained or inexperienced technician introduces another source of measurement error. Similarly, bioelectrical impedance (BIA) has premeasurement guidelines that should be followed, such as no moderate or vigorous exercise 12 hours before testing. If subjects do not adhere to the guidelines, then another source of error is introduced. Each error makes the estimation of body fat less accurate.

Measurement errors cannot be eliminated, but they can be minimized. Athletes should choose the body composition measurement method that is most accurate from among those that are available to them. In many cases body composition estimates provide reasonably accurate and useful information for athletes. However, in some cases the results are too inaccurate to be useful.

Ways to Measure Body Composition

Several methods of measuring body composition are available (see the sidebar for descriptions). As shown in table 10.1, they vary in their accuracy, practicality, availability, and degree of technical expertise needed. Obviously, accuracy would be the primary reason to pick a method if more than one were available. However, many athletes have little choice. Elite athletes can find and afford to have body composition assessed at an imaging center, but a high school athlete may be limited to skinfold measurements. Repeated measurements are needed over time to determine whether body composition goals are being met, so athletes must choose a method that they will have access to repeatedly.

TABLE 10.1   Comparison of Body Composition Measurement Methods

Method	Accuracy*	Practicality and availability	Technical expertise needed
DEXA	SEE = ±1.8%	Imaging centers or university research labs	License required
Underwater weighing	SEE = ±2.7%	Exercise physiology labs and gyms or fitness centers with enough space	Some; not difficult to learn
Bod Pod	SEE = ±2.7-3.7%	Exercise physiology labs, gyms or fitness centers, or offices with enough space	Minimal
Skinfolds	SEE = ±3.5 %	Many settings including exercise physiology labs, training rooms, gyms, or offices	High; proper technique is critical and must be practiced
BIA	SEE = ±3.5%	Many settings including health fairs, gyms, and fitness centers	Minimal
NIR	SEE = ±4%	Many settings including health fairs, gyms, and fitness centers	Minimal

DEXA= dual-energy X-ray absorptiometry; BIA = bioelectrical impedance; NIR = near-infrared interactance

* Based on studies reporting the standard error of the estimate (SEE)

From Dunford/Doyle. *Nutrition for Sport and Exercise*, 1E. © 2008 Brooks/Cole, a part of Cengage Learning, Inc. Reproduced by permission. www.cengage.com/permissions

Interpretation of Body Composition

To prevent giving the false impression that body composition measurements are accurate, results should always be given as a range. For example, if an athlete is underwater weighed and is estimated to be 16 percent body fat, then the athlete should be told that body fat is likely to be between 13.3 and 18.7 percent (SEE = ± 2.7 percent). Additionally, he should be made aware that body composition might be higher or lower than this range. Emphasizing a single number or suggesting that the error of measurement can be overlooked leads to false perceptions.

DESCRIPTION OF VARIOUS BODY COMPOSITION METHODS

- **Air-displacement plethysmography (Bod Pod).** Plethysmography determines body volume by measuring air displacement, which is used to predict body composition. The person sits in an enclosed chamber wearing tight-fitting clothing and a swim cap. This method is quick and easy to perform.

- **Bioelectrical impedance (BIA)**. This method determines body composition by measuring the ability of various tissues, such as fat and water, to conduct electrical currents. Electrodes are typically attached to the wrists and ankles and measurements are made and entered into a prediction equation. This test is simple to perform, but subjects should not eat or drink four hours before, should not consume alcohol 48 hours before, and should not perform moderate physical activity 12 hours before testing.

- **Dual-energy X-ray absorptiometry (DXA, or DEXA)**. In this method, the density of various tissues are measured using low-intensity X-rays. Bone density measurements are especially accurate. Prediction equations are used to estimate body composition. This is one of the most accurate methods at present, but it requires expensive equipment, specialized software to predict body composition, and licensed technicians.

- **Kinanthropometry.** Kinanthropometry involves comprehensive individual measurements of elements that influence movement. It includes measurements of body composition as well as body build and shape. This method emphasizes the accurate measurement of skinfolds over time, which requires a technician with specialized training. The number of trained individuals is small but growing around the world.

- **Near-infrared interactance (NIR)**. Body composition is determined by using a wand to measure tissue absorption or reflection of light. Prediction equations are used to estimate body composition. This method is easy to use, but its accuracy is typically less than that of other methods.

- **Skinfolds**. Calipers are used to measure subcutaneous fat at several (usually three or seven) body sites. An equation is used to estimate body composition, and it is critical to use the most appropriate formula based on ethnicity, sex, and age. It is relatively inexpensive to purchase the calipers, and skinfold measurements may be the only body composition method available at high schools. Because this method is inexpensive and widely available, it is approved for use by most state wrestling associations to determine body composition. A major concern is the error introduced by the technician performing the skinfold measurements. There is an international effort to replace this method with kinanthropometry (described earlier).

- **Underwater (hydrostatic) weighing**. Underwater weighing determines body volume by measuring water displacement. Prediction equations are used to determine body composition. This method requires the subject to stay submerged and still for several seconds while blowing out as much air as possible from the lungs. These requirements are difficult for some people to meet.

There should also be an element of common sense. For example, some highly muscular athletes may have a percentage of body fat that is estimated to be near zero, which is not possible. Similarly, it may be difficult to measure skinfold thickness in some people because the subcutaneous fat layer does not easily separate from the muscle and skin, resulting in an estimate that is too high. Although visual appearance is a highly subjective way to judge body composition, at times the numbers simply do not match the reality. Common sense would suggest that body composition measurements obtained in such cases should be used cautiously.

How Do Weight and Body Composition Relate to Performance?

Elite athletes in a given sport or position tend to be similar in weight and body composition, although they are not exactly the same. It is not possible to precisely predict a percentage of body fat or lean body mass that will result in excellent performance for a given athlete. Changing weight and body composition has the potential to improve an athlete's performance because certain body weights and compositions are well matched to certain sports. As is the case with hydration guidelines, each person must determine, in part by trial and error, optimal performance weight and body composition.

Weight and body composition are influenced by genetic predispositions to leanness and fatness and the distribution of body fat. Any desired changes to weight and body composition must be realistic given the athlete's genetic tendencies. Even if it can be achieved, a body weight or percentage of body fat that is too low may be detrimental to performance because it may be difficult to maintain unless calories and nutrients are routinely restricted. Similarly, too great of a body weight, even if it represents a high percentage of skeletal muscle, may be detrimental because it can decrease **flexibility**, **agility**, or speed. Athletes need to focus on what is both feasible and favorable when setting weight and body composition goals.

flexibility—The ability to bend.

agility—A combination of physical speed, suppleness, and skill.

endurance—The ability to resist fatigue. As a general term, it is more often used in reference to cardiovascular endurance than to muscle endurance.

To determine optimal weight and body composition, an athlete should consider the following:

- The sport and position played
- Size requirements (height and weight) for the sport or position
- Body build (tendency to be thin, muscular, or stocky)
- The relative need for power and **endurance**
- The need for speed, strength, flexibility, agility, and mobility
- The power-to-weight ratio
- The weight certification requirements
- The degree to which body appearance is part of subjective scoring

⭐ SUCCESS STORY

Michelle Rockwell, RK Team Nutrition

Michelle Rockwell, MS, RD, CSSD, is a sport dietitian in private practice (www.rkteamnutrition.com). This is her story:

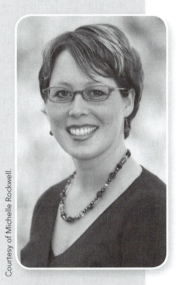

Courtesy of Michelle Rockwell.

"My passion for sport nutrition was born in high school as a member of the soccer and track and field teams. As we strove to enhance performance and reduce body fat (which was measured every three weeks), I distinctly remember a coach advising us to eat less than 15 grams of fat daily. What resulted was talented and motivated high school girls taking this advice to heart—and to the extreme—as we carefully assembled obsessively fat-free diets each day. Not surprisingly, I also remember being very hungry and sore! This was my introduction to the impact of food and nutrition on performance and well-being. I also had a gut feeling that some teammates were taking this well-intended advice too far, which was my firsthand introduction to disordered eating.

"On a recruiting trip as a high school senior, I met Kristine Clark, PhD, RD, the sport nutritionist for Penn State University. I was so impressed by Kris's dedication to health and performance and knew then that working in college sport nutrition was my dream job. I majored in dietetics and exercise science and competed in track and field at Virginia Tech.

"I was hired as the University of Florida's first director of sports nutrition in 1999. I will never forget my first day. I had a legal pad, pen, telephone, and no budget. But I had tremendous support from everyone. I counseled thousands of athletes, created nutrition plans, implemented training table, held hands-on seminars, measured body composition, provided advice on dietary supplements, and coordinated an eating disorder team.

"I relocated to Raleigh-Durham, North Carolina, and started a sport nutrition consulting service. I counsel professional, collegiate, and club-level athletes throughout the United States. I've expanded my practice to include young recreational athletes, casual exercisers, ultraendurance athletes, and Master's competitors. There are so many things that remain the same: I continue to have young female athletes adopting extremely low-fat diets. But so many things have changed, and I thoroughly enjoy keeping up with the latest and greatest of sport nutrition."

Sport Played

In many sports elite athletes tend to be similar in body composition because particular compositions are well matched for the physical demands of particular sports or positions. For example, all elite bodybuilders have a high percentage of skeletal muscle and a low percentage of body fat because that is required to win contests. Elite distance runners tend to have a low percentage of body fat and a low body weight because excess body fat contributes to extra body weight, a mechanical disadvantage when the body needs to be moved quickly and efficiently over a long distance.

Table 10.2 summarizes the results of studies that report the body composition of professional, elite, and collegiate athletes. These studies document the body composition of high-level athletes, but they do not predict the percentage of body fat that will make a given athlete successful. The results are a body fat percentage range for those who have attained success in their sport, so those who aspire to be elite athletes often use these ranges when setting their own goals. Such figures should be used with great caution. Note that the range is large for some sports, such as water polo and tennis, and narrow for others, such as long-distance cycling.

TABLE 10.2   Estimated Body Compositions of Selected Well-Trained Athletes

Sport	Level	Position or distance	% body fat
MALES			
Baseball	College	All positions	11-17
Baseball	Professional	All positions	8.5-12
Basketball	Professional	Centers	9-20
		Forwards	7-14
		Guards	7-13
Cycling, road	Professional	Long distance	7-10
American Football	College (NCAA Division I)	Defensive backs	7-14.5
		Receivers	9-16.5
		Quarterbacks	14-22
		Linebackers	12.5-23.5
		Defensive linemen	14.5-25
		Offensive linemen	18.5-28.5
Judo	National team	All weight classes	8.5-19
Rugby	Professional	All positions	9-20
Soccer	Professional and college	All positions	7.5-18
Tennis	Elite		8-18
Water polo	National team		6.5-17.5
Wrestling	College champions		6.5-16
FEMALES			
Running	Elite	Middle distance	8-16.5
		Long distance	12-18
Soccer	College	All positions	13-19
Swimming or diving	College	Middle distance or diving	17-30
	Masters	Long distance	20-34
Tennis	Elite		15-25

NCAA= National Collegiate Athletic Association

Reprinted, with permission, from M. Macedonio and M. Dunford, 2009, *Athlete's guide to making weight* (Champaign, IL: Human Kinetics), 62.

Weight and body composition are relatively minor factors in some sports. For example, successful professional golfers come in a variety of weights, sizes, and percentages of body fat. Mike Weir, Tiger Woods, and John Daley have very different body compositions, but all have won major golf championships. Similarly, successful baseball or softball pitchers are a variety of sizes and weights. These sports and positions depend to a large degree on fine motor skills and to a much lesser degree on percentage of body fat.

Position Played

Many team sports have a wide range of weights and body compositions among members of the team, but a much narrower range for specific positions. For example, an American football team may have players ranging from 7 to 30 percent body fat, but those at the higher end of the range are almost always linemen. Some additional body fat is beneficial for linemen because opponents have a harder time pushing around bigger players. Similarly, players on rugby and baseball teams vary tremendously in body composition.

Team sports such as basketball, ice hockey, lacrosse, and soccer typically have a smaller range of body fat percentages for the team than American football or rugby because excess body fat is not advantageous in sports that require speed and endurance. However, there are still variations based on the position played. For example, basketball centers tend to have a higher percentage of body fat than small forwards. Although most elite soccer players are lean, those who need relatively more speed and endurance tend to be less muscular and weigh less than other players on the team.

Size

Scientific and anecdotal evidence reveals that athletes today are bigger than their counterparts of the past. One study of professional hockey players of the 1980s and 1990s found that they were approximately 37 pounds (17 kg) heavier and 4 inches (10 cm) taller than their counterparts who played in the 1920s and 1930s, although the percentage of body fat stayed the same (Montgomery, 2006). Currently, several successful women's professional tennis players are 6 feet (183 cm) tall or taller, and today's players are rarely less than 5 feet 5 inches (165 cm) tall. Bigger size confers an advantage in many sports, particularly contact sports, so it is not surprising that the majority of linemen in the National Football League are over 300 pounds (136 kg). Unfortunately, excessive weight and abdominal fat can lead to chronic health problems (Kraemer et al., 2005).

High school and collegiate athletes are bigger than those in the past, and there is a disturbing trend among youth American football players to increase size by increasing fatness (Laurson & Eisenmann, 2007; Malina et al., 2007). Children grow and develop at different ages, so within the same age range there are always children who are taller or larger than others. At an early age a large child who is fat may have an advantage over a smaller child in terms of just physical size. Much of this advantage fades over time, and overfatness becomes a disadvantage when it negatively affects fitness, speed, and health.

An increase in size is often a goal when an athlete steps up to the next level of competition. To successfully compete in college, high school athletes in many sports are expected to get bigger. They need to increase their weight primarily by increasing the amount of skeletal muscle. If collegiate athletes become professionals, then another increase may be expected. An increase in skeletal muscle requires a well-designed resistance training program and a caloric intake sufficient to support the growth of new tissue.

A few sports are extremely size dependent. For example, sumo wrestlers must be large, and ski jumpers must be light in weight because neither can defy the laws of physics. Size is also a factor in wrestling, boxing, rowing, powerlifting, and some of the martial arts. To allow for the participation of more athletes and for fair competition, these sports are divided into weight categories.

Nutrition Bite

Anabolic steroids are tissue-building drugs used by athletes to enhance performance and improve appearance. Athletes who use them typically gain weight and increase muscle size. They may also increase strength and endurance and improve recovery time, features that would theoretically allow them to train harder and improve performance. It is often difficult for athletes to stop using anabolic steroids because of real and perceived changes to body composition, strength, and performance.

The National Strength and Conditioning Association states: "The most important thing that a strength and conditioning coach can do about the problem is to send a clear message to his/her athletes that it is unacceptable to use steroids or growth hormones. This drug problem is a threat to the strength and conditioning coach's very existence. Some athletes think that using anabolic steroids is a substitute for proper training and hard work, and is a shortcut to success . . . . The general public is beginning to assume that all highly successful athletes (especially strength athletes) have achieved success with the aid of anabolic substances. Solutions to the drug problem begin at the high school level or earlier, and coaches at this level are the first line of intervention" (National Strength and Conditioning Association, 2001).

Body Build

Body build, or shape, is influenced by a genetic predisposition to leanness or fatness. In the early 1940s categories based on body shape, known as **somatotypes**, were created. Ectomorphs are thin or slight and have a tendency not to gain large amounts of muscle or body fat. Many elite distance runners are ectomorphs. Mesomorphs have the ability to increase muscle mass substantially but do not easily gain excess body fat. Many elite male bodybuilders are mesomorphs. Endomorphs are typically stocky, and they have a tendency to gain body fat in the abdominal area. Some heavyweight wrestlers are endomorphs, and they often struggle with weight gain, particularly abdominal fat gain, when they discontinue wrestling. Some athletes

somatotype—Body shape, build, and appearance.

fall squarely in one of these three categories, whereas others do not. Knowledge of somatotypes can help an athlete set realistic weight and body composition goals.

Relative Need for Power and Endurance

Each sport can be placed on the power–endurance continuum. At one end is power, the explosive aspect of strength, and at the other end is endurance, prolonged exertion (see figure 10.2). One of the best examples is the 100-meter runner versus the marathon runner. Sprinters need explosive power that is sustained only for seconds, and this is reflected in their size, weight, and body composition. Elite male 100-meter runners are typically tall (over 6 feet, or 183 cm) and weigh around 190 pounds (86 kg), with well-developed upper- and lower-body skeletal muscles and a low percentage of body fat. In contrast, elite male marathon runners are usually shorter than sprinters, weigh considerably less, have less skeletal muscle (although what they have is well developed for distance running), and have a tendency to be light boned. They also have a low percentage of body fat. In each case, the body is well matched for the sport.

Most sports involve varying degrees of power and endurance. For example, soccer, basketball, ice hockey, lacrosse, and tennis require explosive power as well as cardiovascular endurance. Increasing muscle mass and strength is beneficial for increasing explosive power, but an excessive amount of skeletal muscle or body fat is a disadvantage when it decreases endurance or flexibility. These athletes need the proper amount of muscle and fat without having too much or too little, which is clearly a balancing act.

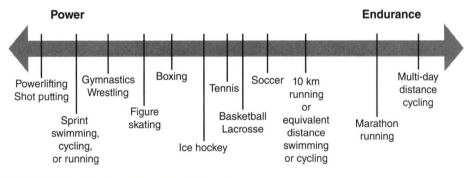

FIGURE 10.2   **Power–endurance continuum.**

Speed, Strength, Flexibility, Agility, and Mobility

In addition to the relative need for power or endurance, athletes must consider the need for speed, strength, flexibility, agility, and mobility and how these must be balanced. For example, basketball players, like sprinters, must be strong and fast runners. However, basketball players must also be flexible, agile, and mobile because they must be able to bend, stretch, and shoot the ball over opposing players. Depending on the position, one or more of these attributes will be emphasized. Centers typically have less mobility than forwards or guards but greater height, size, and strength to score and rebound. Point guards and small forwards must be extremely agile. Typically, centers weigh more and have a larger amount of both fat-free mass and body fat than point guards or small forwards. However, players in each position do vary in terms of weight and body composition.

Speed is critical in many sports. If speed and prolonged cardiovascular endurance are essential, the athlete tends to have a body composition more like an endurance runner than a sprinter. When explosive power (strength and speed but not prolonged endurance) is more critical, the opposite is true. Thus, a striker in soccer has a different weight and body composition than a defender. This is true in many team sports such as American football (receiver versus linebacker), lacrosse (attackman versus defender), and rugby (scrum-half versus prop or hooker).

A few athletes have a primary focus—strength. Examples include powerlifters; shot putters; and hammer, javelin, and discus throwers. These athletes look to increase muscle mass and strength. Speed is not involved, and because they are lifting or throwing an object, some additional body fat may actually be advantageous because it adds to the body's mass (weight). Most athletes cannot be singularly focused because their sports involve a combination of speed, strength, power, endurance, flexibility, agility, and mobility.

> *You need to become more than one type of athlete. You have to be a sprinter, a weight man, and a distance guy all in one.*
>
> **Dan O'Brien**, 1996 Olympic gold medalist in the decathlon and three-time world decathlon champion

Power-to-Weight Ratio

Power-to-weight ratio is defined as power (measured in watts) divided by weight (measured in pounds or kilograms). When the body is moved through space, a high power-to-weight ratio is desirable. In other words, it is a benefit to have a relatively high percentage of muscle mass but no excess body fat because excess fat contributes to dead weight. Dead weight contributes to total weight but does not contribute to muscle power, so it is a disadvantage. Examples of athletes who benefit from a high power-to-weight ratio include high, long, and triple jumpers; distance runners and cyclists; rowers; gymnasts; figure skaters; linebackers; ice hockey players; and wrestlers.

Either an increase in power or a decrease in weight can positively change the power-to-weight ratio. The goal is to have sufficient muscle size and strength but little dead weight. Lesser-trained athletes normally focus first on increasing muscle size and strength, which gives them more power. As they maximize their muscle strength, athletes then put more focus on decreasing dead weight. Athletes typically understand that the reduction of *excess* fat has the potential to improve performance. However, obtaining too low of a percentage of body fat is detrimental to both performance and health and athletes need to understand that fact, too.

Weight Certification Requirements

Weight categories are necessary in some sports because larger athletes would have an unfair advantage over smaller athletes. Because weight must be certified before competition, weight-regulated sports necessarily put considerable emphasis on achieving a particular scale weight. Unfortunately, water can be manipulated to **make weight** because scale weight does not reflect how the composition of the body may have changed. Reduction of water intake, excessive water loss through sweating, and the use of diuretics are ways to temporarily lower body weight. Such manipulations can result in elevated body temperature, which can be dangerous or fatal.

making weight—Being certified to compete in a certain weight category, typically below one's natural weight.

In the past, wrestling represented the dangerous practices used to make weight and cut weight. Rules once allowed wrestlers to weigh in almost one day before a competition and wrestle in any weight category. Many were encouraged to wrestle 10 or 20 pounds (4.5 or 9 kg) below their natural weights, which could only be achieved through dehydration, starvation, excessive exercise, or other extraordinary measures. Wrestling now has rules that require wrestlers to establish a minimum weight category before the beginning of the season based on body composition and proper hydration. For high school and college students these rules are administered by the state wrestling federation and the NCAA, respectively, and can be found on their Web sites. Such rules have been successful in eliminating many of the water weight–related problems of the past. However, not all weight category sports have adopted rule changes that prevent dangerous weight certification practices.

Body Appearance

In some sports the appearance of the athlete's body is considered in the scoring. The best example is bodybuilding, in which the body is the sport. However, athletes in any "artistic" sport or athletic endeavor, such as figure skating, gymnastics, diving,

Nutrition Bite

According to Greek mythology, Adonis was an extremely handsome young man. Today, the Adonis Complex is associated with an obsession by men with obtaining excess muscularity. The medical term is *muscle dysmorphia*. This is considered an obsessive-compulsive disorder, and those suffering from it are encouraged to seek medical and psychiatric attention.

This condition is characterized by a high dissatisfaction with appearance, extreme focus on the amount of skeletal muscle, dependence on weightlifting, frequent checking of body appearance, and frequent thoughts about ways to increase muscularity. A man with this complex may give up all social activities to work out more in the gym or be unwilling to be seen in a bathing suit because he believes his body is not muscular enough. Such thoughts and behaviors put these men at risk for anabolic steroid use (Choi, Pope, & Olivardia, 2002; Kanayama et al., 2006).

cheerleading, and ballet, may be subject to body appearance expectations. These athletes often try to achieve a weight and body composition that match the current cultural norms for the sport because doing so may positively influence the scoring.

In most cases, the expectation for males in artistic sports is a lean, muscular appearance, which is often a consequence of high-volume training. In contrast, the typical expectation for females in these sports (with the exception of bodybuilding) is a thin but not overly muscular appearance. This is harder for many females to achieve and may require chronic undereating. These sports are associated with a higher risk of developing eating disorders in female participants (see chapter 11).

What Is Needed to Increase Muscle Mass?

Simply stated, an increase in skeletal muscle requires a well-designed resistance training program that is supported by a properly formulated dietary program. Although many nutrients are important to muscle growth, the focus is usually on two—calories and protein.

Sufficient calories are needed for muscles to grow. A very rough estimate is that an adult needs to consume an additional 350 to 500 kcal daily above baseline intake to support the manufacture of new muscle tissue. It is usually recommended that males consume an additional 400 to 500 kcal daily and that females consume near the lower end of this range, about 350 kcal more daily.

Most of the additional calories should come from carbohydrate, which is needed to resynthesize the muscle glycogen used for resistance training. Some of the additional calories may also be from protein foods, but increasing calories only by increasing protein consumption can result in carbohydrate intakes that are too low. High-protein, low-carbohydrate diets lead to low muscle glycogen stores after days or weeks of repeated resistance training. Some additional calories may also be consumed in the form of fat. For health reasons these fats should be heart-healthy fats such as nuts, seeds, avocadoes, and oils.

Some additional protein is needed to support the growth of additional skeletal muscle. However, only 22 percent of muscle is protein, so the extra protein required is typically less than most athletes think. Approximately 100 grams of protein is incorporated into each pound (0.5 kg) of new muscle tissue. Assuming a 1-pound increase in skeletal muscle per week, the need for more protein would be about 14 grams per day.

To put the need for additional protein in perspective, 2 ounces (60 grams) of roasted chicken breast provide 14 grams of protein. One scoop (around 33 grams) of protein powder contains approximately 25 grams, similar to the amount found in many protein bars. Thus, most athletes can easily add enough protein to support muscle growth by increasing the portion size of the protein foods they are already consuming or adding one protein-containing food to their daily diets. More information about protein foods and supplements can be found in table 5.2 on page 63.

Many athletes are already consuming high-protein diets, but those who are not could easily alter their dietary intake to add the small amount of protein needed to support skeletal muscle growth. A protein drink, a glass of nonfat milk, or a larger serving of fish would likely do the trick. When the topic is muscle growth, protein intake receives a lot of emphasis; however, overemphasizing protein intake puts the athlete at risk for too low of a carbohydrate intake. Excessive protein intake could also contribute to excess caloric intake, which results in an increase in body fat.

How Much Muscle Mass Can Be Gained?

A male athlete could expect to gain 0.5 to 1.0 pound (0.2 to 0.5 kg) of lean body mass a week. This increase in lean body mass reflects an increase in the protein, water, and glycogen content of the new skeletal muscle. As a very rough estimate, female athletes could expect an increase of 0.25 to 0.75 pound (0.1 to 0.3 kg) of lean body mass a week, about 50 to 75 percent of what males might expect to gain. These figures are only estimates, and athletes vary widely as a result of differences in genetic predisposition and levels of hormones, such as testosterone.

The current state of training must be considered when predicting how much muscle mass an athlete can gain. An untrained person would expect to make considerable gains with a sustained resistance training program supported by a proper diet. A male athlete may experience a 20 percent increase in lean body mass after one year of rigorous resistance training. However, the next year may only result in a 1 to 3 percent increase. Ultimately, there are physical limits to the amount of skeletal muscle a person can gain.

The Short of It

- Body weight and body composition are related to performance, appearance, and health.
- Body weight does not give information about body composition.
- Scale weight is a simple way to estimate hydration status.
- Any measurement of weight or body composition has some degree of error.
- Body composition methods vary in their accuracy, practicality, and availability.
- Optimal weight and body composition depend on the sport or position played, the relative need for strength, running speed, agility, and flexibility, and genetic predisposition to leanness.
- A high power-to-weight ratio is desirable when the body needs to be moved. To increase skeletal muscle size and strength, athletes must follow well-designed resistance training and nutrition programs.
- More calories and protein are needed to build muscle tissue, but the additional amount of protein needed daily is relatively small.

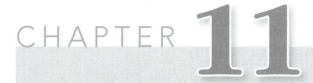

Athletes and Disordered Eating

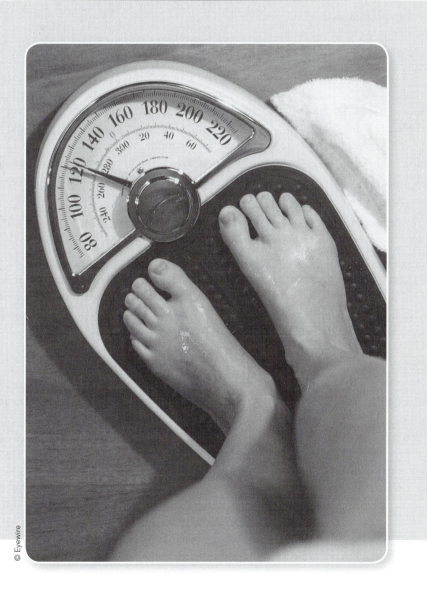

In this chapter, you will learn the following:

✓ How normal eating and disordered eating differ
✓ The criteria for anorexia nervosa and other eating disorders
✓ Sports in which the risk for eating disorders is high
✓ The three conditions that make up the female athlete triad

"When there is no enemy within, the enemies outside cannot hurt you."

African proverb

Although rare, the deaths of elite athletes from eating disorders always cause those involved in sports to pause and wonder what went wrong. How does an elite, Olympic-caliber gymnast who was vibrant at 93 pounds (42 kg) die from complications of anorexia at age 22 weighing less than 60 pounds (27 kg)? And what of those famous athletes who years later reveal their struggles with bulimia? Had no one noticed, or did those with concerns not know how to intervene? How does an off-handed comment about weight by a coach or teammate become the catalyst for eating and exercise behaviors that are ultimately destructive? How does something as normal and pleasurable as eating become so distorted, damaging, and deadly? In the high-pressure world of competitive sports, athletes sometimes begin down a slippery slope from normal eating to eating disorders under cover of darkness (their own and others' lack of knowledge) and are unable to reverse the course of events before it is too late.

How Do Normal and Disordered Eating Differ?

To understand disordered eating, one must first understand normal eating. There is no standard definition for normal eating, but it is both balanced and flexible. For the most part it is eating when hungry and stopping when full, although it is normal to occasionally overeat and undereat. Normal eating involves consuming foods that provide the nutrients the body needs, but eating junk food on occasion is also considered normal. Some constraint is needed, but strictly disciplined or regimented eating is not normal; nor is completely unrestrained eating.

Normal eating for athletes is particularly hard to define. Diet affects training and performance, and athletes generally need to put some focus on their food intake each day. Both overeating and undereating can be detrimental to training and performance, and some dietary discipline is needed for restoring nutrients depleted by rigorous exercise. Some constraint may be necessary for maintaining weight and body composition within an optimal range. Athletes may at times need to be a bit more restrained and disciplined in their eating than nonathletes, but balance and flexibility still apply. Although for athletes normal eating may require discipline, diet should not become an obsession.

disordered eating—A deviation from normal eating.

Disordered eating is a deviation from normal eating and is different than an **eating disorder**. Disordered eating is not as severe as an eating disorder, such as anorexia nervosa. However, a major concern about disordered eating is that it will become more frequent and severe and progress to an eating disorder.

Defining and recognizing disordered eating in athletes can be difficult. First, what is normal eating for an individual athlete must be clear. Then, the degree to which the athlete is deviating from normal must be established. This is particularly hard in athletes because normal eating for an athlete, especially at the elite level, often requires discipline, focus, and mild restraint.

The normal pattern of eating for many low-weight athletes, such as distance runners and female gymnasts, is one of mild restraint of calorie intake. One study found that the daily caloric intake of female endurance and **aesthetic athletes** was approximately 2,400 kcal daily, about 100 kcal less than their estimated energy expenditure (Beals & Manore, 1998). In other words, these females tended to undereat slightly each day. But teammates with disordered eating are also restricting calories. What distinguishes normal from disordered eating in these athletes?

> **eating disorder**—A substantial deviation from normal eating that meets diagnostic criteria established by the American Psychiatric Association.
>
> **aesthetic athletes**—Athletes in sports in which the score is based partly on appearance.

In part, the distinction is based on the severity of the restriction. Undereating by 100 kcal daily is not of the same magnitude as undereating by 300 to 500 kcal daily. There are also differences in focus. The disordered eater likely puts undo focus on scale weight, body appearance, body image, and overly strict discipline. These concerns can lead to less flexibility and balance and to eating-related anxiety. Such athletes may be progressing toward eating disorders.

Table 11.1 on page 153 compares some of the features that distinguish normal eating and exercise behaviors from disordered ones. An athlete's diet should be balanced, flexible, and adequate in calories, but it is only one aspect of life. Athletes with disordered eating patterns can become obsessed with diet, constantly counting

Nutrition Bite

The SCOFF Eating Disorder Quiz was developed and tested at a medical school in London. It is a very simple screening tool for determining who may be at risk for anorexia or bulimia. Each of the five questions should be answered.

1. Do you make yourself **s**ick because you feel uncomfortably full?

2. Do you worry that you have lost **c**ontrol over how much you eat?

3. Have you recently lost more than **o**ne stone (14 lb) in a 3-month period?

4. Do you believe yourself to be **f**at when others say you are too thin?

5. Would you say that **f**ood dominates your life?

One point is awarded for each yes answer. A score of two or more indicates that the individual may be at risk and further assessment is needed. More detailed assessments require specialized training, but this is an excellent initial screening tool that anyone can use.

⭐ **SUCCESS STORY**

Jessica Setnick, Understanding Nutrition and EatingDisorderJobs.com

Drawn to dietetics by the goal of becoming the nutritionist for her hometown Dallas Cowboys, Jessica Setnick, MS, RD, CSSD, ultimately became one of the nation's leading authorities on nutrition counseling for eating disorders.

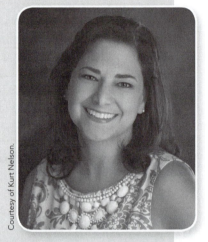

After completing her master's degree in exercise and sport nutrition and two years working on an eating disorders treatment team in a children's hospital, Jessica started her private practice, Understanding Nutrition. As the only nonhospital dietitian in Dallas accepting patients under 14 years old, Jessica quickly became known as the go-to person for children with eating disorders.

Jessica began Eating Disorders Boot Camp—a workshop designed to be "the eating disorders class you never had in school"—as a way for new graduates to gain experience. Eight dietitians attended the first workshop, indicating that it was not only students who needed this crucial information. Swamped with requests for guidance from professionals across the country, Jessica took Eating Disorders Boot Camp on the road, teaching the most current and successful treatment strategies for eating disorders more than 40 times since 2003.

After hearing repeatedly from workshop participants that the Eating Disorders Boot Camp manual was indispensable, Jessica recognized a need for an easy-to-use reference book for treatment professionals. Her self-published *The Eating Disorders Clinical Pocket Guide*, the first book of its kind in the field, was the result. Selling thousands of copies around the world, *The Eating Disorders Clinical Pocket Guide* gained the attention of the American Dietetic Association, who will be publishing the second edition as the *American Dietetic Association Pocket Guide to Eating Disorders*. Jessica's most recent venture is bringing job seekers and job opportunities together via the EatingDisorderJobs.com website.

In her travels for both Eating Disorders Boot Camp and as an invited speaker at conferences and events, Jessica emphasizes the three needs of professionals treating eating disorders—confidence, competence, and community. She says, "Those who work with individuals with disordered eating or eating disorders can feel isolated and wonder if their approaches are appropriate. It is not easy work and progress is often slow. My goal is to provide resources for those who dedicate themselves to helping others overcome eating issues."

how many calories they consume and feeling guilty if they exceed their self-imposed limits. Athletes normally engage in rigorous training but for the purpose of improved performance. Those with disordered eating often overtrain, in part to expend calories so they do not gain any body fat. Overtraining hampers performance and increases the risk of injury.

TABLE 11.1 Comparison of Normal and Disordered Eating Patterns in Athletes

	Normal pattern	**Disordered pattern**
Caloric intake	Daily caloric intake is monitored but not tightly controlled. Amount of calories consumed is adequate.	Daily caloric intake is restricted and tightly controlled and becomes an obsession. Amount of calories consumed is inadequate.
Overall diet	Diet is balanced. Generally healthful foods are consumed, but junk foods are occasionally eaten.	Diet is unbalanced. Foods are categorized as good or bad. Eating "bad" food may cause guilt.
Dietary flexibility	Eating pattern is routine but flexible as needed. Food intake is varied.	Eating pattern is ritualistic and inflexible. Food intake is monotonous.
Body image	Accurate and positive.	Inaccurate and negative. Never satisfied with current body weight or appearance.
Weight and body composition	Well matched for the sport and enhances performance. Goals are attainable without compromising health.	Unrealistic weight and body composition goals that, when met, interfere with training, performance, and health.
Muscle mass	Sufficient muscle mass.	Insufficient muscle mass due to a starvation-type diet.
Training	Exercise is purposeful and focused on improving performance. Overtraining does not occur.	Excessive exercise or voluntary overtraining for the purpose of caloric expenditure.

Athletes with normal and disordered patterns differ, but the differences may be subtle or not evident. For example, an athlete may appear to be running the same number of miles as everyone else on the team. However, unbeknown to the coach, that athlete may also be running on her own. She may eat regularly but only very low-calorie foods, such as green salads. An athlete may be eating the same amount of food at training table as his teammates but may be inducing vomiting within a few minutes after leaving the building.

The eating behaviors of athletes fall on a continuum from normal to extremely abnormal. As is true of any continuum, these behaviors may blend into each other so subtly that it is difficult to know where one starts and another ends. The progression from normal to disordered eating to a full-blown eating disorder is typically gradual and may go unrecognized for a long period of time. Early intervention is key because the chances for successful treatment are much better if behaviors have not been well established.

What Is an Eating Disorder?

An eating disorder is a substantial deviation from normal eating and also involves psychological issues such as body image. The American Psychiatric Association (APA) has defined three distinct eating disorders: anorexia nervosa, bulimia nervosa, and eating disorders not otherwise specified. A fourth condition, anorexia athletica, has been described but is not recognized by the APA as an eating disorder. Diagnostic criteria are listed in the sidebar Diagnostic Criteria for Eating Disorders on page 154.

DIAGNOSTIC CRITERIA FOR EATING DISORDERS

Three distinct eating disorders have been recognized by the American Psychiatric Association (1994).

Anorexia Nervosa

A. Refusal to maintain body weight at or above a minimally normal weight for age and height (e.g., weight loss leading to maintenance of body weight less than 85 percent of that expected; or failure to make expected weight gain during period of growth, leading to body weight less than 85 percent of that expected).

B. Intense fear of gaining weight or becoming fat, even though underweight.

C. Disturbance in the way in which one's body weight or shape is experienced, undue influence of body weight or shape on self-evaluation, or denial of the seriousness of the current low body weight.

D. In postmenarcheal females, amenorrhea (i.e., the absence of at least three consecutive menstrual cycles). (A woman is considered to have amenorrhea if her periods occur only following hormone [e.g., estrogen] administration.)

Specify type:

- Restricting type: During the current episode of Anorexia Nervosa, the person has not regularly engaged in binge-eating or purging behavior (i.e., self-induced vomiting or the misuse of laxatives, diuretics, or enemas).

- Binge-eating/purging type: during the current episode of Anorexia Nervosa, the person has regularly engaged in binge-eating or purging behavior (i.e., self-induced vomiting or the misuse of laxatives, diuretics, or enemas).

Bulimia Nervosa

A. Recurrent episodes of binge eating. An episode of binge eating is characterized by both of the following:

1. Eating, in a discrete period of time (e.g., within any 2-hour period), an amount of food that is definitely larger than most people would eat during a similar period of time and under similar circumstances.

2. A sense of lack of control over eating during the episode (e.g., a feeling that one cannot stop eating or control what or how much one is eating).

B. Recurrent inappropriate compensatory behavior in order to prevent weight gain, such as self-induced vomiting; misuse of laxatives, diuretics, enemas, or other medications; fasting; or excessive exercise.

C. The binge eating and inappropriate compensatory behaviors both occur, on average, at least twice a week for 3 months.

D. Self-evaluation is unduly influenced by body shape and weight.

E. The disturbance does not occur exclusively during episodes of Anorexia Nervosa.

Specify type:

- Purging type: During the current episode of Bulimia Nervosa, the person has regularly engaged in self-induced vomiting or the misuse of laxatives, diuretics, or enemas.

- Nonpurging type: During the current episode of Bulimia Nervosa, the person has used other inappropriate compensatory behaviors, such as fasting or excessive exercise, but has not regularly engaged in self-induced vomiting or the misuse of laxatives, diuretics, or enemas.

Eating Disorders Not Otherwise Specified (EDNOS)

Pathological behaviors are clearly present, but the specific diagnostic criteria for either anorexia nervosa or bulimia nervosa are not met. Examples include:

- For females, all of the criteria for Anorexia Nervosa are met except that the individual has regular menses.
- All of the criteria for Anorexia Nervosa except that, despite significant weight loss, the individual's current weight is in the normal range.
- All of the criteria for Bulimia Nervosa are met except that the binge eating and inappropriate compensatory mechanisms occur at a frequency of less than twice a week or for a duration of less than 3 months.
- The regular use of inappropriate compensatory behaviors by an individual of normal body weight after eating small amounts of food (e.g., self-induced vomiting after the consumption of two cookies).
- Repeatedly chewing and spitting out, but not swallowing, large amounts of food.
- Binge eating disorder: recurrent episodes of binge eating in the absence of the regular use of inappropriate compensatory behaviors characteristic of Bulimia Nervosa.

Anorexia Athletica

Anorexia athletica has been described but is not recognized by the APA as an eating disorder. The following criteria were described by Sudi and colleagues, 2004.

- Reduced body mass (weight) and loss of fat mass is performance related and not related to appearance or body shape. (It should be noted that concerns about body shape could arise as the individual compares body weight, shape, or composition to the sport's most successful athletes.)
- The loss of body mass results in a lean physique.
- Weight cycling (repeated weight gain and loss) is usually present, although maintenance of a low body weight may be seen all year (preseason, competitive season, off-season).
- Restriction of food intake, or excessive exercise, or both are voluntary or at the suggestion of a coach or trainer.
- The abnormal eating occurs while the athlete is competing but stops at the end of the athlete's career.

Anorexia nervosa is characterized by a refusal to maintain body weight, a fear of gaining weight, an extreme distortion of body image, and, in females, **amenorrhea**. The general public most often associates voluntary starvation with anorexia, but some people may also binge eat and purge by vomiting or using laxatives and diuretics. Self-esteem is highly dependent on body weight and self-control. The typical age of onset is 13 to 25 years.

amenorrhea—The absence or suppression of menstruation.

Bulimia nervosa is characterized by binge eating. Some bulimics also purge by vomiting or using laxatives, enemas, and diuretics. Binge eating is stressful, and depression may follow the eating binge. Self-esteem is highly dependent on body weight, body shape, and feelings of being in control. The age of onset can be anywhere from adolescence to middle adulthood.

Eating disorders not otherwise specified are often described as mixed eating disorders because harmful behaviors are present but the criteria for neither anorexia nor bulimia are met. This type of eating disorder is probably the most common, but because it is not well defined, the number of people affected is not known.

Anorexia athletica is driven by performance concerns and is often characterized by weight cycling, which is repeated weight loss and gain. Food is restricted and exercise may be increased beyond that needed for training in an effort to expend additional calories. The athlete can be harmed both physically and psychologically. These eating patterns generally stop when the athlete's career ends. However, there is concern that some former athletes will develop disordered eating behaviors, such as purging, to control weight.

It takes skill and training to recognize and diagnose any of these eating disorders. Certified athletic trainers are often in the best position to detect eating and exercising behaviors that are considered warning signs because they have frequent contact with the athlete. Examples of warning signs include dieting when thin, rigid eating patterns, excessive exercise, and a negative body image. Anyone who has a concern must act as soon as possible by having a person the athlete trusts approach the athlete, express concern, and make a referral to a trained professional. Most college campuses have a confidential referral program in place. If no such program exists, a good starting point is to refer the athlete to a team or primary care physician.

Although intervening can be difficult, worrisome signs and symptoms should not be ignored. The concerned person may want to believe that the athlete will turn

Nutrition Bite

Orthorexia nervosa is an unhealthful obsession with healthful eating. It is ironic that people could become so consumed with the idea of health that their behaviors become unhealthful. The obsession with healthful food, not the quantity of the food consumed or body weight, makes orthorexia different from the eating disorders.

Those with orthorexia consume whole foods with no additives, preservatives, or processing methods that would make the food "impure." Food intake becomes austere and characterized by denial. Social relationships may suffer as they become self-righteous about their diet compared to others.

Obsessive behaviors regarding food are not considered normal. Dietary perfectionism and rigidity often result in nutrient deficiencies because several nutrients, such as vitamins and minerals, depend on a wide variety of foods to provide a sufficient amount. Those with orthorexia would likely benefit from counseling with a psychologist and a registered dietitian with expertise in disordered eating.

things around, but this is wishful thinking in most cases. Athletes do not typically resolve these issues themselves and will need the help of a treatment team. This team typically consists of a physician, psychologist, and dietitian with special training in treating disordered eating. Early intervention is critical because eating disorders can be life threatening.

Which Athletes Are Most Susceptible?

The estimated prevalence of disordered eating and eating disorders ranges from as low as 1.3 percent of the athletic population to as high as 20 percent (Beals, 2006). The least common condition is anorexia nervosa, but it receives much attention because it is a life-threatening disease. Females are more likely to exhibit disordered eating and eating disorders than males. However, males should not be overlooked. The sports that have the highest prevalence are those that favor a low body weight, a low percentage of body fat, or a thin appearance. The following sports are considered high risk for the development of disordered eating and eating disorders

- Bodybuilding
- Horse racing (jockeys)
- Middle- or long-distance running
- Ski jumping
- Swimming
- Weight-class sports, such as boxing, lightweight rowing, martial arts, and wrestling
- Women's aesthetic sports, such as cheerleading, diving, figure skating, and gymnastics

Because these sports have a high prevalence of eating disorders, it is important for coaches, strength and conditioning specialists, certified athletic trainers, teammates, and parents to be aware of eating patterns that deviate from normal. It is important to note that many athletes in these sports have normal eating patterns, just as some athletes in other sports suffer from disordered eating. The sport itself does not cause athletes to develop eating disorders.

Wrestlers may fit the criteria for anorexia athletica, but they typically do not meet the criteria for the other eating disorders. Some wrestlers restrict food and fluids, take diuretics or laxatives, and exercise excessively in an effort to make weight. These wrestlers may eat abnormally during the season, but they are not driven by poor self-esteem or distorted body image. This is a key point because someone with an eating disorder has unresolved psychological issues. Wrestlers in the past were legend in their efforts to make weight, but rule changes by wrestling governing bodies have eliminated many of these harmful practices.

Factors That Influence the Development of Eating Disorders

An eating disorder is a psychiatric disease. However, it does not develop in a vacuum. There are factors that influence the development of disordered eating and eating disorders. These include personality traits, societal norms, and the attitudes of coaches and others who work closely with an athlete.

> *I wanted to be perfect in my attitude and in my weight. Inside I was going crazy. I probably consumed 10,000 calories a day or more in fast foods. I can tell you where every McDonald's and Jack in the Box was along the way (to my voice lessons)—and every bathroom where I could get rid of the food.*
>
> **Cathy Rigby**, in a 1992 *People* magazine article. She was a popular American gymnast in the 1960s and 1970s and spoke out about her eating disorder in the 1980s.

Several personality traits are associated with the development of eating disorders. These include perfectionism, obsessive-compulsive behavior, and the need to attain a goal at any cost. This is not to say that anyone with these traits will develop an eating disorder. However, these traits are highly valued in athletics, and athletes receive positive reinforcement for exhibiting them. In the context of an eating disorder, which is a psychiatric disease, the traits that receive positive feedback may be the same traits that are making the disease worse.

Western society's body image norms for women are often mentioned as a factor in the increase in the number of cases of eating disorders since the 1960s. The media tend to emphasize thin females and dieting. Females who equate thinness with success are more likely to develop eating disorders. Female athletes can face enormous pressures about their appearance, with some athletes being called out in the press for gaining body fat.

No one person can cause an eating disorder in someone else. However, coaches have tremendous influence on their athletes, and a coach's opinion may be more highly valued by an athlete than anyone else's opinion. Therefore, an International Olympic Committee (IOC) Medical Commission report specifically recommends that coaches not be involved in any way in changing an athlete's weight or body composition.

Unfortunately, many coaches are involved in the athlete's weight-related issues, and this makes it trickier for them. Coaches may inadvertently pressure an athlete to achieve a weight or percentage of body fat that is not appropriate. For example, it may appear to a coach that a 190-pound (86 kg) female volleyball player could easily lose 10 pounds (4.5 kg), but this may not be desirable or possible if she already has a low percentage of body fat. Coaches may also make comments about weight loss that are incorrect or misinterpreted by the athlete. A thin distance runner may hear her coach joke about the "thunder thighs" of one of the female shot-putters. If this runner has an inaccurate body image, she may believe that her own thighs are too big and that the coach is also directing the comment to her. Therefore, coaches must be cautious when talking about weight or body composition.

> *There's a lot of mixed messages being sent. On one page, a person who is normal is overweight, the next page, someone who's skinny is anorexic. You have to have a sense of self and worth to make sure you don't get swayed by the bad influences out there.*
>
> **Anna Kournikova,** a former professional tennis player, answering the question "What do you tell kids you work with about body image?" Kournikova was known as much for her looks as for her tennis.

What Is the Female Athlete Triad?

The female athlete triad involves three interrelated factors: energy availability, menstrual function, and bone mineral density (BMD). Each of these factors is highly influenced by both diet and exercise. Each factor develops along a spectrum from optimal to dysfunctional as shown in figure 11.1. Ideally, each female athlete would have optimal energy availability, normal menstruation, and optimal bone health. Unfortunately, female athletes may develop low energy availability, disrupted menstrual function, and low bone mineral density. Each of these conditions is detrimental, and because they are interrelated they can have far-reaching effects on the athlete's health.

Energy availability refers to how well caloric intake is matched with energy expenditure and is an important factor in the triad. When caloric intake is substantially and persistently below what is needed for performing exercise training, then normal body functions are affected. Low energy availability may be the result of disordered eating or an eating disorder. However, it may be due to inadvertently eating too few calories. For example, an athlete may lack appetite after rigorous training, and sleeping may be a higher priority than eating. Low energy availability may also be a result of intentionally eating too few calories in an effort to keep from gaining weight. Regardless of the cause, low energy availability forces the body to adapt to a persistent semistarvation state, which results in hormonal imbalance and other problems.

Menstrual function is another factor in the triad. Menstrual hormones, such as estrogen and **luteinizing hormone**, are affected by low energy availability. Athletes may be anywhere on the menstrual function spectrum from normal

luteinizing hormone—One of the hormones involved in ovulation.

menstruation, known as eumenorrhea, to intermittent menstruation to amenorrhea, a lack of menstruation. Low estrogen also negatively affects bone mineral density, the third component of the triad. Low bone mineral density is a risk factor for developing osteoporosis. Although osteoporosis is most often associated with women over age

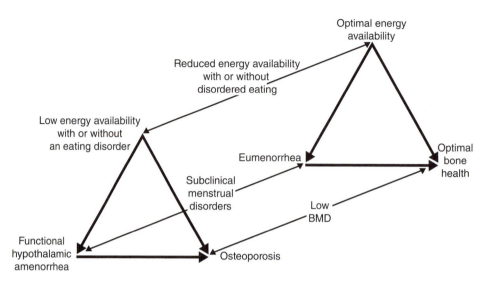

FIGURE 11.1 The female athlete triad. The spectrums of energy availability, menstrual function, and bone mineral density along which female athletes are distributed (narrow arrows). An athlete's condition moves along each spectrum at a different rate, in one direction or the other, according to her diet and exercise habits. Energy availability, defined as dietary energy intake minus exercise energy expenditure, affects bone mineral density both directly via metabolic hormones and indirectly via effects on menstrual function and thereby estrogen (thick arrows).

Reprinted by permission from American College of Sports Medicine, 2007. "The female athlete triad," *Medicine and Science in Sports and Exercise* 39(10), 1868.

50, it can develop in athletes at a young age. Some female athletes, such as long-distance runners, have been diagnosed with osteoporosis in their mid- to late-20s. The three factors in the triad move from optimal to less optimal to dysfunctional within different time frames, so it is possible that an athlete with low energy availability has not yet developed one of the obvious dysfunctional conditions, such as lack of menstruation.

Screening for the female athlete triad should be part of a female athlete's physical exam. Although any female can be at risk for low energy availability, menstrual dysfunction, and low bone mineral density, distance runners, ballet dancers, swimmers, gymnasts, and lightweight rowers are known to be at higher risk because low weight is a factor in appearance and performance. The reversal of low energy intake is important for the athlete's health. If calories are being restricted because of disordered eating, then the athlete should be referred to treatment, including psychotherapy, because the reasons for restricting food intake may be deep-seated and not easily resolved. A sport dietitian can help an athlete develop strategies to match food intake with energy expenditure even on busy training days. Menstrual irregularities and low bone mineral density are medical problems that need treatment by a physician. Further information about the female athlete triad can be found in the American College of Sports Medicine or the IOC position stands.

The Short of It

- The keys to normal eating and a healthful diet are moderation, balance, and flexibility.
- Disordered eating and eating disorders are deviations from normal eating that lead to psychological and medical problems.
- Although females are most often affected by disordered eating and eating disorders, males should not be overlooked.
- Eating disorders can be fatal, and intervention should not be delayed.
- All female athletes should be screened for the triad.
- Low energy availability, disrupted menstrual hormones, and loss of bone mineral density, alone or in combination, are detrimental to the athlete's health and need treatment.

The Future of Sport and Exercise Nutrition

The future of sport and exercise nutrition is bright. There have been tremendous advances in knowledge and its application, particularly in the last 15 years, and more advances are expected. The number of full-time jobs is slowly increasing. Athletes at all levels are looking seriously at the role nutrition plays in training, recovery, and performance. As athletes compete at the professional level for longer periods of time than in the past, nutrition becomes particularly important because of its role in recovery and good health. Although no one can predict the future with accuracy, some likely developments in the field of sport and exercise nutrition are outlined here.

Job Opportunities

The number of full-time jobs in sport nutrition is expected to slowly increase. A major issue is credentialing and the distinction between sport nutritionists and sport dietitians. In the United States, there is no requirement for people who work in the field of sports nutrition to be licensed. Thus, individual employers set the qualifications for the job. At the present time, the strongest credential in terms of education and experience appears to be the board-certified specialist in sports dietetics (CSSD), which requires that the person be a registered dietitian.

Dual Areas of Expertise

Most athletes would benefit from the expertise of a sport dietitian. Unfortunately, budgets at the high school and club levels are usually small and strained, so it is beyond the budget to hire such a person. Being certified in two areas, such as sport dietetics and strength and conditioning, could be beneficial because there may be enough money in the budget for a full-time person who is qualified to work in both areas.

Entrepreneurial Skills

An entrepreneur is someone who sets up and finds financing for new commercial enterprises. The field of sport and exercise nutrition is ripe for entrepreneurs. New forms of communication such as video conferencing, text messaging, and social networking Web sites may provide the platform for some creative ways to counsel athletes about nutrition.

Nutrigenomics

Nutrigenomics is the use of genetic information to determine the specific nutrients and type of diet a person needs to prevent disease. Scientists have already shown that specific nutrients as well as general dietary patterns can influence genes. Therefore, one of the forefronts in the field of nutrition is creating personalized diets based on a person's unique genetic makeup.

Genetic testing can identify variant genes, which are slightly different from the usual form of genes. The difference can be very small; for example, only one of the hundreds of building blocks of the gene may be different. Variant genes are not necessarily bad. However, some can contribute to disease states or undesirable health outcomes.

One of the best examples of nutrigenomics comes from studies of a variant gene that affects the metabolism of folic acid. People with this variant gene are at higher risk for heart disease and stroke. Those who have the variant gene benefit from a daily folic acid supplement (Stover & Caudill, 2008).

Some genetic variations already discovered may be of particular interest for athletes. For example, three variant genes associated with antioxidant activity have been identified. A link between caffeine and bone loss has been discovered, but only if one particular variant gene is present. Several variant genes are known to be pro-inflammatory, and this response can be offset to some degree by eating oily fish or supplementing with fish oil. There are also variant genes associated with abnormal levels of blood sugar and insulin (Arkadianos et al., 2007).

In the future, athletes may be genetically tested, and physicians and sport dietitians may use the information to tailor diets that reflect specific variant gene–nutrient interactions. An individualized plan can be created, and that plan may include the use of vitamin or mineral supplements as medications. Nutrigenomics, or personalized nutrition, is likely the wave of the future.

Molecular Biology and Sport Nutrition

When we think of nanotechnology, we think of things being very small. Computers, telephones, and other communications devices have been revolutionized by nanotechnology. It is likely that sport nutrition will be revolutionized by the study of the human body at the smallest level, which is the molecular level.

One of the biggest breakthroughs in sport nutrition came with the study of muscle cells in the late 1960s. These studies were conducted at the cellular level and yielded new information about muscle glycogen. The ability to maximize the amount of carbohydrate stored in muscle cells by adopting a high-carbohydrate diet proved to be one of the most important discoveries for athletes. Today, scientists in the fields of nutrition and exercise physiology are also looking at changes at the molecular level. For example, they study specific enzymes in muscle cells associated with the metabolism of muscle glycogen. These studies yield very specific information about cellular processes that, in turn, may be applied to athletes to improve training, recovery, or performance. For example, studies of enzymes in muscle cells led to recommendations about nutrient timing.

It is hoped that molecular biology will better our understanding of protein metabolism. Protein is one of the more difficult nutrients to study in the body because it is found throughout the body and it is hard to measure small changes in protein status. In particular, athletes are interested in maximizing muscle growth and minimizing muscle damage from resistance exercise. Ultimately, scientists will understand protein synthesis and breakdown on the molecular level, which will lead to more specific recommendations about the amount, type, and timing of protein intake for athletes.

Keeping Up With New Knowledge

Nutrition and exercise physiology are evolving fields. Part of the responsibility of a sport-related professional is keeping up-to-date with the newest recommendations. Thus, continuing education is not only necessary, it is imperative.

One way to stay abreast of new developments is to attend conferences. Organizations such as the American College of Sports Medicine (ACSM), American Dietetic Association (ADA), National Strength and Conditioning Association (NSCA), and National Athletic Trainers' Association (NATA) feature nutrition lectures and workshops at their annual meetings. These forums also give participants a chance to ask questions directly of the speaker.

There has been tremendous growth of online offerings in the area of sport nutrition. University courses offer comprehensive coverage of the subject. Professional organizations and companies, such as Human Kinetics, also offer numerous self-study courses. Online courses are convenient and beneficial, but interactivity may be limited.

Journal articles are very important in the dissemination of knowledge. Some are review articles, which summarize the most recent information about a topic. Other articles report the results of new studies. These articles offer more specific information about a subject, but the reader must incorporate this information into the body of knowledge about that topic. The National Library of Medicine Online (PubMed) is a free search engine that anyone can use to access the database containing the article citations. In some cases, the full text of the article is available free of charge, but more often only the abstract is available.

Appendix A

Learn More About Sport and Exercise Nutrition

Books

▶ Beals, K. (2004). *Disordered eating among athletes*. Champaign, IL: Human Kinetics.

Comprehensive guide for health professionals. In-depth coverage of a very complicated topic.

▶ Dunford, M., & Doyle, J.A. (2008). *Nutrition for sport and exercise*. Belmont, CA: Thomson/Wadsworth.

College textbook designed for undergraduates. Comprehensive coverage of all topics relevant to sport nutrition.

▶ Macedonio, M., & Dunford, M. (2009). *The athlete's guide to making weight*. Champaign, IL: Human Kinetics.

A guide to determining and achieving optimal performance weight. Guides athletes and those who work with them through a program that can help them change weight and body composition.

▶ Seebohar, B. (2005). *Nutrition periodization for endurance athletes: Taking traditional sports nutrition to the next level*. Boulder, CO: Bull Publishing.

Matches nutrition with training for endurance athletes. Written by a sport dietitian formerly employed by the U.S. Olympic Training Center who is an ultraendurance athlete himself.

▶ Wilmore, J.H., Costill, D.L., & Kenney, W.L. (2008). *Physiology of sport and exercise*, 4th ed. Champaign, IL: Human Kinetics.

College exercise physiology textbook. Comprehensive coverage of the physiology of sport and exercise.

Journal Articles

▶ American Dietetic Association, Dietitians of Canada, & the American College of Sports Medicine: Nutrition and athletic performance (position paper). (2009). *Journal of the American Dietetic Association, 109,* 509-527. Also printed in *Medicine & Science in Sports & Exercise, 41,* 709-731.

Joint position paper by experts of all three organizations outlining the latest evidence-based information about nutrition as it relates to athletic performance.

▶ American College of Sports Medicine, Armstrong, L.E., Casa, D.J., Millard-Stafford, M., Morna, D.S., et al. (2007). American College of Sports Medicine position stand. Exertional heat illness during training and competition. *Medicine & Science in Sports and Exercise, 39,* 556-572.

Position paper written by experts in the field of heat illness and athletes. Guidelines are evidence based.

▶ American College of Sports Medicine, Sawka, M.N., Burke, L.M., Eichner, E.R., Maughan, R.J., et al. (2007). American College of Sports Medicine position stand. Exercise and fluid replacement. *Medicine & Science in Sports and Exercise, 39,* 377-390.

Position paper written by experts in the field of fluid replacement. Emphasizes individual application of evidence-based guidelines.

▶ National Athletic Trainers' Association position statement: Preventing, detecting, and managing disordered eating in athletes. (2008). *Journal of Athletic Training, 43,* 80-108.

Excellent resource for certified athletic trainers and others who interface with athletes. Gives practical information about disordered eating and what concerned people can do.

▶ Phillips, S.M., Moore, D.R., & Tang, J.E. (2007). A critical examination of dietary protein requirements, benefits, and excesses in athletes. *International Journal of Sport Nutrition and Exercise Metabolism, 17,* 608-623.

A discussion of protein as it relates to athletes.

▶ Sacks, F.M., Bray, G.A., Carey, V.J., et al. (2009). Comparison of weight-loss diets with different compositions of fat, protein, and carbohydrates. *New England Journal of Medicine, 360,* 859-873.

Results of a well-designed research study that addresses the question, Which weight loss diet is best?

▶ Volek, J.S., & Rawson, E.S. (2004). Scientific basis and practical aspects of creatine supplementation for athletes. *Nutrition, 20* (7-8), 609-614.

Summarizes the numerous research studies conducted on creatine supplements in athletes.

Web Sites

▶ American College of Sports Medicine. www.acsm.org

Promotes and integrates scientific research, education, and practical applications of sports medicine and exercise science including sport nutrition.

▶ Ask the Sports Dietitian at *Runner's World.* http://askthesportsdietitian.runnersworld.com

Twice-monthly column written by a sport dietitian.

▶ Sports, Cardiovascular, and Wellness Nutrition. www.scandpg.org

A practice group of the American Dietetic Association. Includes information about becoming a board-certified specialist in sport dietetics.

▶ Sports Dietitians Australia. www.sportsdietitians.com.au

Professional organization of dietitians specializing in sport nutrition. Also provides information about nutrition for athletes.

Appendix B

Implementing Sport and Exercise Nutrition in the Real World

Athlete

☐ Learn as much as you can about how nutrition affects training, recovery, and athletic performance.

☐ Assess your current diet and compare it to the guidelines recommended for athletes. The most accurate dietary assessments are those conducted by a sport dietitian.

☐ Determine the usual weight and body composition of successful athletes in your sport. Assess your body composition and the genetic potential for you to change the amount of muscle and fat you currently have. Consult with someone well trained in body composition assessment, such as an exercise physiologist.

☐ Use the assessment information to set weight and body composition goals that are appropriate for you.

☐ Set clear goals and objectives, such as the amount of muscle mass to be gained or the amount of body fat to be lost. Set a realistic time frame, recognizing that you can gain or lose ~1 pound (0.5 kg) of fat per week.

☐ Determine the amount of calories, carbohydrate, protein, and fat needed each day based on your training plan.

☐ Translate the amount of nutrients needed to specific foods and beverages that contain those nutrients. Plan meals and snacks. A sport dietitian can help create a nutrition program just for you and help you determine whether you need to take supplements.

☐ Assess your daily hydration status by weighing yourself before and after exercise and looking at the color of your urine. Create a plan for obtaining enough fluid daily.

☐ Reassess your plans periodically to make sure you are making progress toward your goals.

Physician

☐ Encourage athletes to eat a healthful diet regardless of the purpose of their appointment.

☐ Ask questions about behaviors that may be detrimental to the athlete such as anabolic steroid use, a large and rapid loss of weight, or the use of dietary supplements.

☐ Screen for any nutrient deficiencies, such as iron-deficiency anemia.

☐ Screen for any nutrition-related health problems such as high blood pressure, elevated blood lipids, elevated blood glucose, or the accumulation of truncal fat. Help athletes see the connection between a good diet and good health.

☐ Screen for the female athlete triad.

☐ Be aware that some athletes struggle with disordered eating behaviors and that such behaviors can get worse and lead to eating disorders such as anorexia or bulimia. Use the SCOFF or another screening tool to identify those at risk. Once identified, counsel the athletes or refer them to a psychologist.

☐ Although most eating disorders occur in females, don't overlook the males. Pay special attention to sports in which low body weight is advantageous, such as ski jumping, horse racing (jockeys), and distance running. In females, be aware of the sports that have a high incidence and prevalence of eating disorders, such as gymnastics, figure skating, and ballet.

Head or Assistant Coach

☐ Set an example by following a healthful diet yourself. "Do as I say not as I do" sends a mixed message about the importance of diet to training, performance, and health.

☐ Focus on the improvement of training and performance by encouraging athletes to attain an optimal performance weight and body composition. However, designate others to work directly with the athlete on these issues. If available, refer the athlete to the sport dietitian for long-term counseling.

☐ Encourage athletes to follow sport nutrition guidelines by making it convenient for them to do so. For example, athletes are more likely to rehydrate if fluid is available. Similarly, nutritious snacks after exercise help athletes to recover. However, there may be rules that prohibit providing food for athletes.

☐ Support the use of training table so that athletes may eat nutritious meals together.

☐ Be aware of the potential for disordered eating and eating disorders. Become familiar with the protocols for referral and treatment at your institution. If there are no protocols, insist that the institution develop them.

☐ If you suspect that an athlete is struggling with food-related issues, refer the athlete immediately for help. Do not try to counsel the athlete yourself. Special training is needed to work with those with psychologically driven negative eating or exercise behaviors.

☐ Recognize that problems with weight, body composition, and eating can be very sensitive for the athlete. Consider this confidential information. Do not share with teammates or make statements to the press about these issues.

Strength and Conditioning Specialist

☐ Set an example by following a healthful diet yourself. "Do as I say not as I do" sends a mixed message about the importance of diet to training, performance, and health.

☐ Strength and conditioning specialists provide guidance regarding nutrition because it is an integral part of increasing muscle mass and supporting training and conditioning. However, many athletes will need more than general sport nutrition information. Providing ongoing nutrition counseling is beyond the scope of practice for strength and conditioning specialists and takes time away from your primary area of expertise. Refer athletes who need nutrition assessments, comprehensive nutrition plans, and nutrition counseling to a sport dietitian.

☐ Do not tell athletes that they should eat a certain way because that strategy has worked for you. It is appropriate to say that your favorite way to get carbohydrate is by eating lots of brown rice. It is inappropriate to tell the athlete that he must eat brown rice.

☐ Take continuing education classes in the area of sport nutrition to make sure that your guidance is up-to-date.

☐ Be aware of the potential for disordered eating and eating disorders. Become familiar with the protocols for referral and treatment at your institution. If there are no protocols, insist that the institution develop them.

☐ If you suspect that an athlete is struggling with food-related issues, refer the athlete immediately for help. Do not try to counsel the athlete yourself. Special training is needed to work with those with psychologically driven negative eating or exercise behaviors.

Certified Athletic Trainer

☐ Set an example by following a healthful diet yourself. "Do as I say not as I do" sends a mixed message about the importance of diet to training, performance, and health.

☐ Certified athletic trainers provide guidance regarding nutrition because it is an integral part of athletic performance and can help to prevent injuries. However, many athletes will need more than general sport nutrition information. Providing ongoing nutrition counseling is beyond the scope of practice for certified athletic trainers and takes time away from your primary area of expertise. Refer those athletes who need nutrition assessments, comprehensive nutrition plans, and nutrition counseling to a sport dietitian.

☐ Take continuing education classes in the area of sport nutrition to make sure that your guidance is up-to-date. The National Athletic Trainers' Association offers many opportunities for continuing education in this area, including online courses.

☐ Remind athletes of the importance of proper hydration on a daily basis. Easy access to a scale encourages athletes to take their weight before and after exercise.

☐ As a certified athletic trainer, you must be aware of the potential for disordered eating and eating disorders. You are often the first person the athlete talks to about eating problems. Therefore, you must be familiar with the protocols for referral and treatment at your institution. If there are no protocols, insist that the institution develop them.

☐ If you suspect that an athlete is struggling with food-related issues, refer the athlete immediately for help. Do not try to counsel the athlete yourself. Special training is needed to work with those with psychologically driven negative eating or exercise behaviors.

Exercise Physiologist

☐ Learn as much as you can about how nutrition affects training, recovery, and performance.

☐ Work closely with other professionals because the athlete benefits from a team approach. For example, an exercise physiologist, sport dietitian, and certified strength and conditioning coach make an excellent team.

☐ Focus on collaboration rather than competition with sport-related personnel. For example, you can be responsible for measuring and establishing body composition goals with the athlete. Collaborate with the strength and conditioning specialist about the training and conditioning program needed to achieve these goals. Both of you can also collaborate with the sport dietitian about a nutrition program that supports the athlete's training, conditioning, and body composition objectives.

☐ Team up with a sport dietitian to give presentations to coaches and athletes. In many cases you will explain the principles behind the recommendations, and the sport dietitian will give the details of an eating plan. For example, you can describe how muscles use carbohydrate and the importance of daily carbohydrate intake to restore muscle glycogen. The sport dietitian can describe the foods that contain carbohydrate and the types of meals and snacks needed to provide the proper amount and timing of carbohydrate intake.

Fitness Professional or Personal Trainer

☐ Set an example by following a healthful diet yourself. "Do as I say not as I do" sends a mixed message about the importance of diet to fitness and health.

☐ Do not tell clients that they should eat a certain way because that strategy has worked for you. It is appropriate to say that your favorite breakfast is yogurt and whole-wheat toast. It is inappropriate to tell your client that this is the best breakfast or that he should eat this way too.

☐ Give general nutrition guidance that has been well documented by scientific studies. For example, emphasize the importance of eating fruits, vegetables, and whole grains daily.

☐ Help people to make general changes in their dietary intake rather than specific changes. For example, talk about consuming an appropriate portion size, eating when hungry and stopping when full, or including more vegetables daily. Refer clients who need in-depth counseling to a dietitian.

☐ Recognize that a basic healthful diet is sufficient for the majority of people who are trying to improve their fitness. Athletes who engage in near-daily training have an increased need for carbohydrate and protein, but most people do not train rigorously enough to fall into this category.

☐ Help people set realistic goals for weight loss. People are not likely to lose more than 1 or 2 pounds (0.5 or 0.9 kg) a week. Large, rapid losses of weight achieved through starvation diets are not likely to be maintained. In fact, many people regain the weight lost.

☐ Slow, sustained weight loss requires a high degree of motivation, and clients need an ever-enthusiastic cheerleader.

☐ Emphasize that people who are fit can get all the nutrients they need from their diets. Supplements are not necessary for most people.

☐ Give clients unbiased advice. If you sell a product or supplement, then your advice is not unbiased. Always inform your client if you will be financially rewarded if they buy a product from you.

Sport Program Administrator

☐ Encourage good nutrition at every level of the program, including your own staff meetings.

☐ Support programs that encourage athletes to eat well. For example, training table gives athletes access to nutritious foods in a team setting.

☐ Demonstrate the program's commitment to healthful foods by having them available for sale. For example, stock vending machines with bottled water, low-fat chocolate milk, apples, or small bags of carrot sticks. These foods can be sold at a profit.

☐ Consider the cost–benefit ratio rather than just the cost when reviewing the budget. High-sugar, high-fat foods often cost less than nutritious foods, but the benefit from nutritious foods is high.

☐ Recognize that nutrition-related features of your program, such as access to working with a sport dietitian or training table, are good recruiting tools especially with freshman athletes and their parents.

☐ If you do not have a protocol for the identification and treatment of eating disorders in place, then establish one immediately. Several universities have well-established programs and are willing to share their protocols and their experiences.

☐ If you suspect or hear that potentially dangerous practices are occurring, investigate them. For example, if rumor has it that some athletes are taking supplements that contain banned substances, don't ignore them. Supplement samples can be tested in an independent lab.

Appendix C

Abbreviations, Acronyms, and Conversions

Abbreviations

c = cup

C = Celsius

Ca = calcium

Cal or C = Calorie

cal or c = calorie

CHO = carbohydrate

cm = centimeter

d = day

F = Fahrenheit

g = gram

hr = hour

in = inch

kcal = kilocalorie

kcal/g = kilocalories per gram

kcal/kg = kilocalories per kilogram of body weight

kg = kilogram

km = kilometer or kilometre

L = liter

lb = pound

m = meter

mcg or μg = microgram

mg = milligram

Mg = magnesium

min = minute

ml = milliliter

oz = ounce

tbsp = tablespoon

tsp = teaspoon

Acronyms

ACE = American Council on Exercise

ACSM = American College of Sports Medicine

AFPA = American Fitness Professionals & Associates

AFTA = American Fitness Training of Athletics

ATC = Certified athletic trainers

BIA = Bioelectrical impedance

BMI = Body Mass Index

CISSN = Certified Sports Nutritionist—International Society of Sports Nutrition

CSCS = Certified Strength and Conditioning Specialist

CSSD = Board Certified Specialist in Sports Dietetics

DXA or DEXA = Dual-Energy X-ray Absorptiometry

IFPA = International Fitness Professionals Association

IOC = International Olympic Committee

NATA = National Athletic Trainers' Association

NFPT = National Federation of Professional Trainers

NIR = Near-infrared interactance

NSCA = National Strength and Conditioning Association

RD = Registered dietitian

SEE = Standard Error of the Estimate

Equivalents and Conversions

Weight

1 oz = 28.35 g or ~ 30 g

1 lb = 0.45 kg

1 kg = 2.2 lb

55 kg = 121 lb

70 kg = 154 lb

90 kg = 198 lb

110 kg = 242 lb

Volume

1 US fluid oz = ~30 ml

2 oz = ~60 ml

4 oz = ~120 ml

8 oz = ~240 ml

Distance

1 inch = 2.5 cm

1 foot = 30.5 cm

1 yard = 91 cm

1 cm = 0.4 inch

1 m = 3 feet 3 inches

1 mile = 1.6 km

1 km = 0.62 mile

Temperature

Celsius = 0.555 × (°Fahrenheit − 32)

Fahrenheit = (°Celsius × 1.8) + 32

20 °C = 68 °F

25 °C = 77 °F

26.7 °C = 80 °F

30 °C = 86 °F

35 °C = 95 °F

37 °C = 98.6 °F

37.8 °C = 100 °F

40 °C = 104 °F

45 °C = 113 °F

Bibliography

American College of Sports Medicine position stand. (2007). The female athlete triad. *Medicine & Science in Sports & Exercise, 39,* 1867-1882.

American College of Sports Medicine, Armstrong, L.E., Casa, D.J., Millard-Stafford, M., Morna, D.S., et al. (2007a). American College of Sports Medicine position stand. Exertional heat illness during training and competition. *Medicine & Science in Sports & Exercise, 39,* 556-572.

American College of Sports Medicine, Sawka, M.N., Burke, L.M., Eichner, E.R., Maughan, R.J., et al. (2007b). American College of Sports Medicine position stand. Exercise and fluid replacement. *Medicine & Science in Sports & Exercise, 39,* 377-390.

American Dietetic Association, Dietitians of Canada, & the American College of Sports Medicine: Nutrition and athletic performance (position paper). (2009). *Journal of the American Dietetic Association, 109,* 509-527.

American Dietetic Association. (2007). Board certification as a specialist in sports dietetics. Retrieved June 18, 2009, from www.cdrnet.org/certifications/spec/sports.htm.

American Heart Association Nutrition Committee, Lichtenstein, A.H., Appel, L.J., Brands, M., Carnethon, M., et al. (2006). Diet and lifestyle recommendations revision 2006: A scientific statement from the American Heart Association Nutrition Committee. *Circulation, 114,* 82-96.

American Psychiatric Association. (1994). Eating disorders. In *Diagnostic and Statistical Manual of Mental Disorders,* 4th ed. (DSM-IV). Washington, DC: American Psychiatric Publishing, Inc., pp. 539-550.

Arkadianos, I., Valdes, A.M., Marinos, E., Florou, A., Gill, R.D., et al. (2007). Improved weight management using genetic information to personalize a calorie controlled diet. *Nutrition Journal, 6,* 29.

Armstrong, L.E., Costill, D.L., & Fink, W.J. (1985). Influence of diuretic-induced dehydration on competitive running performance. *Medicine & Science in Sports & Exercise, 17,* 456-461.

Baker, L.B., Conroy, D.E., & Kenney, W.L. (2007). Dehydration impairs vigilance-related attention in male basketball players. *Medicine & Science in Sports & Exercise, 39,* 976-983.

Baker, L.B., Dougherty, K.A., Chow, M., & Kenney, W.L. (2007). Progressive dehydration causes a progressive decline in basketball skill performance. *Medicine & Science in Sports & Exercise, 39,* 1114-1123.

Baum, A. (2006). Eating disorders in the male athlete. *Sports Medicine, 36,* 1-6.

Beals, K.A. (2006). Disordered eating in athletes. In Dunford, M. (ed.), *Sports nutrition: A practice manual for professionals.* Chicago: American Dietetic Association, pp. 336-354.

Beals, K.A., & Manore, M.M. (1998). Nutritional status of female athletes with subclinical eating disorders. *Journal of the American Dietetic Association, 98,* 419-425.

Beals, K.A., & Manore, M.M. (2002). Disorders of the female athlete triad among collegiate athletes. *International Journal of Sport Nutrition and Exercise Metabolism, 12,* 281-293.

Beard, J., & Tobin, B. (2000). Iron status and exercise. *American Journal of Clinical Nutrition, 72* (2 Suppl.), 594S-597S.

Beck, B.R., & Snow, C.M. (2003). Bone health across the lifespan—exercising our options. *Exercise and Sport Sciences Reviews, 31,* 117-122.

Bergstrom, J., Hermansen, L., & Saltin, B. (1967). Diet, muscle glycogen, and physical performance. *Acta Physiologica Scandinavica, 71,* 140-150.

Bjelakovic, G., Nikolova, D., Gluud, L.L., Simonetti, R.G., & Gluud, C. (2007). Mortality in randomized trials of antioxidant supplements for primary and secondary prevention. *Journal of the American Medical Association, 297,* 842-857.

Bossu, C., Galusca, B., Normand, S., Germain, N., Collet, P., et al. (2007). Energy expenditure adjusted for body composition differentiates constitutional thinness from both normal subjects and anorexia nervosa. *American Journal of Physiology: Endocrinology and Metabolism, 292,* E132-E137.

Burke, L.M., Kiens, B., & Ivy, J.L. (2004). Carbohydrates and fat for training and recovery. *Journal of Sports Sciences, 22,* 15-30.

Cheuvront, S.N., & Sawka, M.N. (2005). Hydration assessment of athletes. *Sports Science Exchange,* 97 (Suppl.), 2.

Choi, P.Y., Pope, H.G., Jr., & Olivardia, R. (2002). Muscle dysmorphia: A new syndrome in weightlifters. *British Journal of Sports Medicine, 36,* 375-377.

Cobb, K.L., Bachrach, L.K., Greendale, G., Marcus, R., Neer, R.M., et al. (2003). Disordered eating, menstrual irregularity, and bone mineral density in female runners. *Medicine & Science in Sports & Exercise, 35,* 711-719.

Coggan, A.R., Raguso, C.A., Gastaldelli, A., Sidossis, L.S., & Yeckel, C.W. (2000). Fat metabolism during high-intensity exercise in endurance-trained and untrained men. *Metabolism, 49,* 122-128.

Cook, C.M., & Haub, M.D. (2007). Low-carbohydrate diets and performance. *Current Sports Medicine Reports, 6,* 225-229.

Corrigan, B., & Kazlauskas, R. (2003). Medication use in athletes selected for doping control at the Sydney Olympics (2000). *Clinical Journal of Sport Medicine, 13,* 33-40.

Costill, D.L., Bowers, R., Branam, G., & Sparks, K. (1971). Muscle glycogen utilization during prolonged exercise on successive days. *Journal of Applied Physiology, 31,* 834-838.

Cox, G.R., Broad, E.M., Riley, M.D., & Burke, L.M. (2002). Body mass changes and voluntary fluid intakes of elite level water polo players and swimmers. *Journal of Science and Medicine in Sport, 5,* 183-193.

Coyle, E.F. (2004). Fluid and fuel intake during exercise. *Journal of Sports Sciences, 22,* 39-55.

Cribb, P.J., Williams, A.D., Stathis, C.G., Carey, M.F., & Hayes, A. (2007). Effects of whey isolate, creatine, and resistance training on muscle hypertrophy. *Medicine & Science in Sports & Exercise, 39,* 298-307.

Dulloo, A.G., & Jacquet, J. (1998). Adaptive reduction in basal metabolic rate in response to food deprivation in humans: A role for feedback signals from fat stores. *American Journal of Clinical Nutrition, 68,* 599-606.

Dunford, M., & Doyle, J.A. (2008). *Nutrition for sport and exercise.* Belmont, CA: Thomson/Wadsworth.

Ebert, T.R., Martin, D.T., Bullock, N., Mujika, I., Quod, M.J., et al. (2007). Influence of hydration status on thermoregulation and cycle hill climbing. *Medicine & Science in Sports & Exercise, 39,* 323-329.

Edwards, A.M., Mann, M.E., Marfell-Jones M.J., Rankin, D.M., Noakes, T.D., et al. (2007). Influence of moderate dehydration on soccer performance: Physiological responses to 45 min of outdoor match-play and the immediate subsequent performance of sport-specific and mental concentration tests. *British Journal of Sports Medicine, 41,* 385-391.

Ganio, M.S., Casa, D.J., Armstrong, L.E., & Maresh, C.M. (2007). Evidence-based approach to lingering hydration questions. *Clinics in Sports Medicine, 26,* 1-16.

Gleeson, M., Nieman, D.C., & Pedersen, B.K. (2004). Exercise, nutrition and immune function. *Journal of Sports Science, 22,* 115-125.

Grandjean, A.C. (1997). Diets of elite athletes: Has the discipline of sports nutrition made an impact? *Journal of Nutrition, 127* (5 Suppl.), 874S-877S.

Gropper, S.S., Smith, J.L., & Groff, J.L. (2005). *Advanced nutrition and human metabolism.* Belmont, CA: Thomson/Wadsworth.

Harp, J.B., & Hecht, L. (2005). Obesity in the National Football League. *Journal of the American Medical Association, 293,* 1061-1062.

Harris, W.S. (2007). Omega-3 fatty acids and cardiovascular disease: A case for omega-3 index as a new risk factor. *Pharmacological Research, 55,* 217-223.

Hawley, J.A. (2002). Effect of increased fat availability on metabolism and exercise capacity. *Medicine & Science in Sports & Exercise, 34,* 1485-1491.

Howarth, K.R., Moreau, N.A., Phillips, S.M., & Gibala, M.J. (2009). Co-ingestion of protein with carbohydrate during recovery from endurance exercise stimulates skeletal muscle protein synthesis in humans. *Journal of Applied Physiology, 106,* 1394-1402.

Institute of Medicine. (1997). Dietary Reference Intakes for calcium, phosphorus, magnesium, vitamin D and fluoride. Food and Nutrition Board. Washington, DC: The National Academies Press.

Institute of Medicine. (1998). Dietary Reference Intakes for thiamin, riboflavin, niacin, vitamin B_6, folate, vitamin B_{12}, pantothenic acid, biotin and choline. Food and Nutrition Board. Washington, DC: The National Academies Press.

Institute of Medicine. (2000). Dietary Reference Intakes for vitamin C, vitamin E, selenium and carotenoids. Food and Nutrition Board. Washington, DC: The National Academies Press.

Institute of Medicine. (2001). Dietary Reference Intakes for vitamin A, vitamin K, arsenic, boron, chromium, copper, iodine, iron, manganese, molybdenum, nickel, silicon, vanadium, and zinc. Food and Nutrition Board. Washington, DC: The National Academies Press.

International Olympic Committee (IOC) Working Commission Working Group Women in Sport. (2005). Position stand on the female athlete triad. Retrieved June 18, 2009 from http://multimedia.olympic.org/pdf/en_report_917.pdf.

International Society of Sports Nutrition. (2008). CISSN: Certified sports nutritionist. Retrieved June 18, 2009 from www.sportsnutritionsociety.org/cert_cissn.aspx.

Ivy, J.L., Katz, A.L., Cutler, C.L., Sherman, W.M., & Coyle, E.F. (1988). Muscle glycogen synthesis after exercise: Effect of time of carbohydrate ingestion. *Journal of Applied Physiology, 64,* 1480-1485.

Jeukendrup, A. (2007). Carbohydrate supplementation during exercise: Does it help? How much is too much? *Gatorade Sports Science Institute,* SSE #106. Retrieved October 6, 2008, from www.gssiweb.com/Article_Detail.aspx?articleid=757&level=2&topic=15.

Kanayama, G., Barry, S., Hudson, J.I., & Pope, H.G., Jr. (2006). Body image and attitudes toward male roles in anabolic-androgenic steroid users. *American Journal of Psychiatry, 35,* 283-291.

Kraemer, W.J., Torine, J.C., Silvestre, R., French, D.N., Ratamess, N.A., et al. (2005). Body size and composition of National Football League players. *Journal of Strength and Conditioning Research, 19,* 485-489.

Laurson, K.R., & Eisenmann, J.C. (2007). Prevalence of overweight among high school football linemen. *Journal of the American Medical Association, 297,* 363-364.

Layman, D.K., Evans, E., Baum, J.I., Seyler, J., Erickson, D.J., et al. (2005). Dietary protein and exercise have additive effects on body composition during weight loss in adult women. *Journal of Nutrition,* 135, 1903-1910.

Leenders, N.Y., Sherman, W.M., & Nagaraja, H.N. (2006). Energy expenditure estimated by accelerometry and doubly labeled water: Do they agree? *Medicine & Science in Sports & Exercise, 38,* 2165-2172.

Leenders, N.Y., Sherman, W.M., Nagaraja, H.N., & Kien, C.L. (2001). Evaluation of methods to assess physical activity in free-living conditions. *Medicine & Science in Sports & Exercise, 33,* 1233-1240.

Legal drug running. (2002, September 28). *The Sydney Morning Herald.*

Lucas, C.J.P. (1905). *The Olympic Games, 1904.* St. Louis, MO: Woodard & Tiernan.

Lukaski, H. (2000). Magnesium, zinc, and chromium nutriture and physical activity. *American Journal of Clinical Nutrition, 72* (Suppl.), 585S-593S.

Lukaski, H.C. (2004). Vitamin and mineral status: Effects of physical performance. *Nutrition, 20,* 632-644.

Macedonio, M., & Dunford, M. (2009). *The athlete's guide to making weight.* Champaign, IL: Human Kinetics.

Magkos F., & Yannakoulia, M. (2003). Methodology of dietary assessment in athletes: Concepts and pitfalls. *Current Opinion in Clinical Nutrition and Metabolic Care, 6,* 539-549.

Malczewska, J., Raczynski, G., & Stupnicki, R. (2000). Iron status in female endurance athletes and in non-athletes. *International Journal of Sport Nutrition and Exercise Metabolism, 10,* 260-276.

Malina, R.M., Morano, P.J., Barron, M., Miller, S.J., Cumming, S.P., et al. (2007). Overweight and obesity among youth participants in American football. *Journal of Pediatrics, 151,* 378-382.

Mathieu, J. (2005). What is orthorexia? *Journal of the American Dietetic Association, 105,* 1510-1512.

Maughan, R.J. (2005). Contamination of dietary supplements and positive drug tests in sport. *Journal of Sports Science, 23,* 883-889.

McDowall, J.A. (2007). Supplement use by young athletes. *Journal of Sports Science and Medicine, 6,* 337-342.

Montgomery, D.L. (2006). Physiological profile of professional hockey players—A longitudinal comparison. *Applied Physiology, Nutrition, and Metabolism, 31,* 181-185.

National Athletic Trainers' Association. (2008). Position statement: Preventing, detecting, and managing disordered eating in athletes. *Journal of Athletic Training, 43,* 80-108.

National Strength and Conditioning Association. (2001). Combating anabolic steroid abuse. Retrieved June 18, 2009, from www.nsca-lift.org/Publications/combating.pdf.

National Strength and Conditioning Association. (2007). About the CSCS credential. Retrieved June 18, 2009, from www.nsca-cc.org/cscs/about.html.

Nelson, J.L., & Robergs, R.A. (2007). Exploring the potential ergogenic effects of glycerol hyperhydration. *Sports Medicine, 37,* 981-1000.

Noakes, T.D., Sharwood, K., Speedy, D., Hew, T., Reid, S., et al. (2005). Three independent biological mechanisms cause exercise-associated hyponatremia: Evidence from 2,135 weighed competitive athletic performances. *Proceedings of the National Academy of Sciences, 102,* 18550-18555.

Peake, J.M. (2003). Vitamin C: Effects of exercise and requirements with training. *International Journal of Sport Nutrition and Exercise Metabolism, 13,* 125-151.

Phillips, S.M., Moore, D.R., & Tang, J.E. (2007). A critical examination of dietary protein requirements, benefits, and excesses in athletes. *International Journal of Sport Nutrition and Exercise Metabolism, 17,* 608-623.

Poortmanns, J.R., & Dellalieux, O. (2000). Do regular high protein diets have potential health risks on kidney function in athletes? *International Journal of Sport Nutrition and Exercise Metabolism, 10,* 28-38.

Rankin, J.W. (2002). Weight loss and gain in athletes. *Current Sports Medicine Reports, 1,* 208-213.

Sacks, F.M., Bray, G.A., Carey, V.J., et al. (2009). Comparison of weight-loss diets with different compositions of fat, protein, and carbohydrates. *New England Journal of Medicine, 360,* 859-873.

Seebohar, B. (2006). Nutrition for endurance sports. In Dunford, M. (ed.), *Sports nutrition: A practice manual for professions.* Chicago: American Dietetic Association, pp. 445-459.

Sherman, W.M., Costill, D.L., Fink, W.J., & Miller, J.M. (1981). Effect of exercise and diet manipulation on muscle glycogen and its subsequent use during performance. *International Journal of Sports Medicine, 2,* 114-118.

Sherman, W.M., Doyle, J.A., Lamb, D.R., & Strauss, R.H. (1993). Dietary carbohydrate, muscle glycogen, and exercise performance during 7 d of training. *American Journal of Clinical Nutrition, 57,* 27-31.

Sports, Cardiovascular and Wellness Nutrition, a dietetic practice group of the American Dietetic Association. (2008). Sports nutrition education programs. Retrieved February 23, 2009, from www.scandpg.org/sport_nutrition_education_program.php.

Steigler, P., & Cunliffe, A. (2006). The role of diet and exercise for the maintenance of fat-free mass and resting metabolic rate during weight loss. *Sports Medicine, 36,* 239-262.

Stover, P.J., & Caudill, M.A. (2008). Genetic and epigenetic contributions to human nutrition and health: Managing genome-diet interactions. *Journal of the American Dietetic Association, 108,* 1480-1487.

Sudi, K., Ottl, K., Payerl, D., Baumgartl, P., Tauschmann, K., et al. (2004). Anorexia athletica. *Nutrition, 20,* 657-661.

Thompson, J. & Manore, M.M. (1996). Predicted and measured resting metabolic rate of male and female endurance athletes. *Journal of the American Dietetic Association,* 96(1), 30-34.

Tipton, K.D., & Wolfe, R.R. (2004). Protein and amino acids for athletes. *Journal of Sports Sciences, 22,* 65-79.

Tipton, K.D., Elliott, T.A., Cree, M.G., Wolf, S.E., Sanford, A.P., & Wolfe, R.R. (2004). Ingestion of casein and whey proteins result in muscle anabolism after resistance exercise. *Medicine & Science in Sports & Exercise, 36,* 2073-2081.

Torstveit, M.K., & Sundgot-Borgen, J. (2005). The female athlete triad: Are elite athletes at increased risk? *Medicine & Science in Sports & Exercise, 37,* 184-193.

Urso, M.L., & Clarkson, P.M. (2003). Oxidative stress, exercise, and antioxidant supplementation. *Toxicology, 189,* 41-54.

van der Merwe, P.J., & Grobbelaar, E. (2005). Unintentional doping through the use of contaminated nutritional supplements. *South African Medical Journal, 95* (7), 510-511.

Van Itallie, T.B., & Nufert, T.H. (2003). Ketones: Metabolism's ugly duckling. *Nutrition Reviews, 61,* 327-341.

Venkatraman, J.T., & Pendergast, D.R. (2002). Effect of dietary intake on immune function in athletes. *Sports Medicine, 32,* 323-340.

Volek, J.S., & Rawson, E.S. (2004). Scientific basis and practical aspects of creatine supplementation for athletes. *Nutrition, 20* (7-8), 609-614.

Volek, J.S., Forsythe, C.E., & Kraemer, W.J. (2006). Nutritional aspects of women strength athletes. *British Journal of Sports Medicine, 40,* 742-748.

Volpe, S.L. (2007). Micronutrient requirements for athletes. *Clinics in Sports Medicine, 26,* 119-130.

Williams, S.L., Stobel, N.A., Lexis, L.A., & Coombes, J.S. (2006). Antioxidant requirements of endurance athletes: Implications for heath. *Nutrition Reviews, 64,* 93-108.

Wilmore, J.H., Costill, D.L., & Kenney, W.L. (2008). *Physiology of sport and exercise*, 4th ed. Champaign, IL: Human Kinetics.

Index